MANUAL OF GERIA

Already published

Cardiology *K. D. Dawkins*
Chest Medicine *J. E. Stark, J. E. Shneerson, T. Higenbottam and C. D. R. Flower*
Child Development *S. Lingam and D. R. Harvey*
Clinical Blood Transfusion *B. Brozovic and M. Brozovic*
Community Paediatrics *L. Polnay*
Gynaecology *T. R. Varma*
Gastroenterology *B. T. Cooper and M. J. Hall*
Haematology *A. Baughn, A. Hughes, K. Patterson and L. Stirling*
Hospital Paediatrics *G. Hambleton*
Medical Procedures *M. J. Ford, C. E. Robertson and J. F. Munro*
Renal Diseases *C. B. Brown*
Rheumatology *J. M. H. Moll*

MANUAL OF GERIATRIC MEDICINE

T. J. M. Van der Cammen
MD
Consultant Physician in Geriatric Medicine
University Hospital Dijkzigt;
Senior Lecturer,
Erasmus University,
Rotterdam, The Netherlands

G. S. Rai
MD MSc FRCP
Consultant Physician in Geriatric Medicine,
Whittington and Royal Northern Hospitals,
London; Senior Lecturer,
University College and Middlesex School of Medicine, London, UK

A. N. Exton-Smith
CBE MA MD DM(Hon) FRCP
Emeritus Professor of Geriatric Medicine,
University of London; Consultant Adviser,
Geriatric Neurophysiology Unit,
Whittington Hospital, London, UK

with a contribution by
Sava Soucek
MD PhD
Consultant in Audiological Medicine,
St Mary's Hospital/Central Middlesex Hospital;
Honorary Senior Lecturer, St Mary's Hospital Medical School,
University of London, London, UK

Churchill Livingstone

EDINBURGH LONDON MELBOURNE AND NEW YORK 1991

CHURCHILL LIVINGSTONE
Medical Division of Longman Group UK Limited

Distributed in the United States of America by Churchill Livingstone Inc., 1560 Broadway, New York, N.Y. 10036, and by associated companies, branches and representatives throughout the world.

First published 1991

ISBN 0-443-03433-8

British Library Cataloguing in Publication Data
Van der Cammen, T. J. M.
    Manual of geriatric medicine.
    1. Geriatrics
    I. Title   II. Rai, G. S.   III. Exton-Smith, A. N.
    618.97

Produced by Longman Singapore Publishers (Pte) Ltd.
Printed in Singapore.

PREFACE

One of the greatest challenges in medical practice today is the care of the increasing number of elderly patients presenting to family doctors as well as specialists. The health care needs of the ageing population differ substantially from those of younger patients. The physical, social and psychological changes associated with ageing are often combined with the debilitating effects of multiple, often co-existing, acute and chronic disease. Both the presentation of disease and the response to treatment are altered in old age and special knowledge is required to deal with these problems.

Although in the last few years teaching in geriatric medicine has increased at undergraduate and postgraduate levels, many medical students and junior medical staff have limited contact with clinicians practising in geriatric medicine. Consequently, they may lack the capacity to assess adequately elderly patients and to provide appropriate health care for them.

This book has been written to provide a practical, problem-orientated approach to common medical problems in the elderly, for family doctors as well as house officers and specialists. The book provides readily available information for them, distinguishing physiological age-related changes from pathological processes and offering guidelines for treatment. It is envisaged that the book would be useful also for doctors preparing for the Royal College of Physicians' Diploma Examination in Geriatric Medicine. It is also hoped that the book will find its way on to the bookshelves of many hospital libraries, both in the UK and in other countries, so that the information in it will be of help to medical students and hospital doctors, who see so many elderly patients in their daily practice.

T. J. M. Van der Cammen
G. S. Rai
A. N. Exton-Smith

ACKNOWLEDGEMENTS

Figures 2.1, 2.2, 2.3 and 2.4 are taken from Johnstone M. 1978 Restoration of motor function in the stroke patient. Churchill Livingstone, Edinburgh by permission of the publishers.

Figure 5.1 is from Rossor M. N. 1982 Neurotransmitters and CNS disease: Dementia. Lancet 2: 1422 by permission of Martin Rossor and The Lancet.

Figure 5.2 is from Bergmann K. 1982 in Magnussen G. et al (eds) Epidemiology and prevention of mental illness in old age. EGV, Hellerup, Denmark.

Figure 8.1 is from Moser M. 1988 Physiological differences in the elderly. In: Boxton R. (ed) Risk factor modification in the elderly. European Heart Journal 9: 55–61 by permission of the Editor of the European Heart Journal.

Figure 23.1 is from Wintrobe et al (eds) 1974 Harrison's principles and practice of medicine, 7th edn. McGraw-Hill, New York and originally from Homans 1945 A textbook of surgery. Charles C. Thomas, Springfield, Illinois, courtesy of the publishers.

Figure 30.1 is reproduced by permission of K. Siersbaeck-Nielsen and The Lancet.

Table 9.2 is from Bayer et al 1986 in the Journal of the American Geriatrics Society 34(4): 263–266 by permission of the author and the American Geriatrics Society.

Tables 24.1 and 24.2 are from Caird F. I. 1985 in Exton-Smith N., Weksler M. E. (eds) Practical geriatric medicine. Churchill Livingstone, Edinburgh by permission of the author and the publishers.

Other acknowledgements have been made at the appropriate place in the text. In the event of an acknowledgement having been inadvertently overlooked, the publishers should like to be informed so that they can insert the necessary information at the first opportunity.

CONTENTS

1. STROKE

Definition

Stroke is an episode of neurological dysfunction lasting for more than 24 hours, caused by a vascular event in the brain. It is usually focal, but may be global, as in subarachnoid haemorrhage.

Epidemiology

— In the UK approximately 100 000 people per year suffer a first stroke. The incidence increases rapidly with age; the annual age-adjusted incidence for the UK is approximately 2 strokes per 1000
— Aneurysmal subarachnoid haemorrhage affects approximately 1 in 10 000 of the population per year. It can occur at any age but is very rare under 10 years of age, and uncommon under 20 years of age. Typically, it is a condition of middle age (i.e., 40–60 years of age) and affects women more than men in a ratio of 3:2
— Half of all first strokes occur in people aged 75 years and over
— Stroke is the cause of one in eight deaths and forms a burden of disability and misery for patients and their carers

Pathogenesis

Causes of stroke
— Cerebral infarction (due to either arterial thrombosis or embolism): approximately 80% of cases
— Primary intracerebral haemorrhage: approximately 10% of cases
— Subarachnoid haemorrhage: approximately 5% of cases
— Unknown factors: approximately 5% of cases

Cerebral infarction
Occurs when an artery is occluded in the absence of an adequate collateral circulation. Occlusion may be due to arterial thrombosis, embolism from proximal arterial thrombi or embolism from the heart.

Primary intracerebral haemorrhage

Bleeding is usually due to either the rupture of a berry aneurysm, an arteriovenous malformation (often leading to bleeding into the subarachnoid space) or hypertensive vascular disease (with bleeding into the brain tissue). Other causes of primary intracerebral haemorrhage are: rupture of small vascular malformations, thrombocytopenia, coagulation disorders and the use of anticoagulants, inflammatory arterial disease, mycotic aneurysms in bacterial endocarditis.

Subarachnoid haemorrhage

This is a haemorrhage into the subarachnoid space, originating from a ruptured berry aneurysm at the base of the brain, or from an angioma or arteriovenous malformation on the brain surface.

Precipitating factors

Hypertension is the most important risk factor for both primary intracerebral haemorrhage and cerebral infarction. The risk of cerebral infarction rises with increasing levels of either systolic or diastolic blood pressure. Other risk factors for cerebral infarction are: age, cardiac disease, especially atrial fibrillation, mitral and aortic valve abnormalities, endocarditis, myocardial infarction with presumed mural thrombus, diabetes mellitus, transient ischaemic attack, high plasma fibrinogen.

— Possible risk factors for cerebral infarction are: cigarette smoking, hyperlipaemia, high haematocrit

Clinical manifestations

Symptoms and signs of a stroke depend on the location and extent of the infarction or haemorrhage or ischaemia. It is not always clear whether the carotid or the vertebrobasilar arterial supply is involved. Hemiparesis, hemisensory loss, dysarthria and even hemianopia can occur in both carotid and vertebrobasilar ischaemia. A large infarction or haemorrhage impairs consciousness wherever the lesion is located. Cerebral thrombosis, embolism and haemorrhage cause a sudden neurological deficit, which may worsen with time ('stroke-in-evolution') due to:

- Further thrombosis or embolization
- Continuing haemorrhage
- Haemorrhagic infarction
- Occurrence of cerebral oedema around the area of the infarction or haemorrhage

Development of associated oedema usually results in a gradual deterioration over 48 hours.

Acute neurological deficit may improve rapidly if there is little neuronal damage, for example when an embolus disintegrates or only a very small infarction or haemorrhage has occurred.

On the other hand, the deficit may be so large it may lead to death within 1–2 days.

Subarachnoid haemorrhage
The patient typically presents with severe generalized headache; neck stiffness is always present, but may be absent in the first few hours after onset of bleeding; hemiparesis may occur a few days after onset of bleeding and is due to cerebral vasospasm; lumbar puncture will show blood or xanthochromia if it is done after a few hours; suspected subarachnoid haemorrhage is an indication for CT scan of the brain; establishing the diagnosis is important because of the implication of surgical management. Subarachnoid haemorrhage has a high mortality: 50% of patients who suffer a subarachnoidal haemorrhage will die of the initial or of a repeat haemorrhage.

Lacunar infarcts
Small (up to 1.5 cm in diameter), deep infarcts, often multiple, usually located in the basal ganglia or the pons. They cause weakness and/or sensory loss down one side of the body; in addition, dysarthria or ataxia may occur. They do not impair cognitive function or cause hemianopia or loss of consciousness. Causal factor is supposed to be the presence of hypertensive changes in the small perforating arteries of the internal capsule, basal ganglia and brain stem.

Transient global amnesia
A clinical syndrome: for several hours, the patient cannot remember recent events, and does not know where he is; long-term memory is intact; possible causes are epilepsy, migraine and ischaemia within the distribution of the posterior cerebral arteries supplying the brain's limbic system. Often a cause is never found.

Multi-infarct dementia
A single stroke may cause impairment of memory and intellect, and a succession of minor vascular events can sometimes lead to multi-infarct dementia. Deterioration is usually 'stepwise' (see also Ch. 5).

Border zone infarction (watershed infarction)
This condition may cause visual disorientation or cortical blindness, and is often associated with a visual field deficit and memory impairment. The causal factor is impairment of cerebral perfusion, for instance due to a sudden fall in blood pressure.

Cerebellar haematoma
The patient with this treatable condition presents with sudden headache, unsteadiness, a rapid reduction in consciousness and brain stem signs, particularly a gaze palsy to the side of the lesion. Suspected cerebellar haematoma is an indication for CT scan of the brain since evacuation of the blood can lead to marked improvement.

Differential diagnosis

The following conditions may be misdiagnosed as a stroke
— Intracranial tumour
— Subdural haematoma
— Meningitis
— Encephalitis
— Hypoglycaemia
— Hyperosmolar diabetic coma
— Side effects of drugs
— Psychogenic factors (neuroses)

Subdural haematoma

This condition should be suspected in patients whose level of consciousness fluctuates over a number of days and who also demonstrate a hemiparesis; it is often associated with a history of trauma to the head but this is present quite often in patients with cerebral infarction or haemorrhage because they fall.

Differentiation between **cerebral infarction** or **intracerebral haemorrhage** is necessary when anticoagulant or other antithrombotic therapy is considered; CT scanning must be done within 2 weeks of onset (i.e. before any primary intracerebral haemorrhage has disappeared). CT scanning is invaluable in diagnosing the cause of a stroke.

Identification of a **cardiac source of embolism** is important because anticoagulation may possibly protect patients with intracardiac thrombus from further embolism; accurate identification can be difficult because both cardiac and arterial sources of embolism may coexist in the same patient.

Complications of stroke

Local

1. Further thrombosis or embolization
2. Continuing haemorrhage
3. Haemorrhage into an infarcted area (haemorrhagic infarction)
4. Development of oedema around the infarction or haemorrhage increases the space-occupying effect of the lesion, and thus the risk of transtentorial herniation and secondary brain stem haemorrhage

All four increase morbidity and mortality.

5. Focal or generalized epilepsy is an uncommon complication, occurring in less than 10% of patients, either acutely or in the long term

General complications

1. Pulmonary embolism
2. Bronchopneumonia, particularly if swallowing and gag reflex mechanisms are impaired

3. Deep venous thrombosis, especially of the paralysed leg
4. Dehydration
5. Pressure sores
6. 'Frozen shoulder' in patients with upper limb paralysis
7. Contractures in spastic limbs
8. Urinary tract infection
9. Urinary incontinence
10. Constipation
11. Falls and injuries
12. Depression/anxiety/personality changes

Investigations

Aims
1. To confirm clinical diagnosis
2. To determine a possible underlying treatable cause
3. To determine risk factors which may be manipulated to prevent recurrence
4. To establish a baseline from which improvement or deterioration can be measured

Investigations include
— ESR
— Full blood count including platelet count
— Plasma lipids
— Serum glucose level
— Urea and electrolytes
— Serum creatinine level
— Urine examination
— Chest X-ray (on indication)
— ECG
— Echocardiography (on indication)
— CT scan (on indication)

Indication for echocardiography
When there is a strong clinical suspicion of cardiac embolic stroke and anticoagulation or other specific treatment is considered.

Indications for CT scan
— Uncertain diagnosis of stroke
— Contemplated anticoagulant or other antithrombotic therapy
— Suspected cerebellar haematoma
— Suspected subarachnoid haemorrhage
— Possible endarterectomy in the future

Information CT scan can give
— CT scan can confirm intracerebral haemorrhage within minutes of onset if the collection of blood is more than 0.5 cm in diameter, or if there is blood in the ventricles or in substantial quantities in the subarachnoid space. Blood

which is evident on the CT scan can completely disappear within 2 weeks
— CT scan can confirm cerebral infarcts larger than approximately 0.5 cm in diameter, but they take 1–2 days to appear and often disappear after 3–4 weeks before reappearing again about 6 months after the stroke
— A low-density area on the CT scan several weeks after a stroke may be caused by a previous haemorrhage or infarct. Brain stem lesions are more difficult to detect than supratentorial lesions

Management

The early management of a stroke involves maintenance of airway in an unconscious patient, maintenance of hydration and nutrition, and care of the bowel, bladder and skin.
— There is no place for drug treatment of acute stroke
  • Small randomized trials have suggested that some drugs (i.e. glycerol, naftidrofuryl, nimodipine) may be effective in limiting the neuronal damage associated with stroke; however, there is insufficient evidence to justify the use of these drugs outside large randomized trials
  • Reduction of oedema surrounding the infarction or haemorrhage has been attempted with glycerol and dexamethasone; again there is no convincing evidence of benefit
  • Low molecular weight dextran has been given IV for its effect on plasma volume and platelet behaviour; it was found to reduce immediate but not late mortality in severe stroke and to have no effect on functional recovery
  • Despite the fact that some vasodilators will increase cerebral blood flow, there is no convincing evidence that they are of value for patients after a stroke
— Surgery plays a limited role in the treatment of acute stroke. A neurosurgical opinion should be sought immediately for patients with a subarachnoid haemorrhage who are considered suitable candidates for surgery
  • Other indications for surgery in selected patients are a cerebellar haematoma or a haematoma situated superficially in the temporal lobe

Aims of management
1. To treat underlying disease
2. To prevent and to treat general complications (chest physiotherapy, good nursing care)
3. To start rehabilitation as soon as possible
4. To manipulate risk factors to prevent recurrence
— There is strong scientific evidence that antiplatelet treatment

for ischaemic stroke reduces recurrence, and aspirin is
recommended in a dose of 300 mg daily

— It has not been established that the incidence of a
recurrence of embolization in patients with cardiac disease
can be reduced by anticoagulation therapy. Anticoagulation
may be considered for patients with ischaemic stroke
associated with atrial fibrillation, cardiac valve disease or
myocardial infarction with presumed mural thrombus,
provided there is no evidence of haemorrhage on the CT
scan. In addition, opinions vary as to when treatment
should be commenced. Some advocate a delay of treatment
for 3 weeks to reduce the risk of haemorrhagic infarction,
while others start treatment immediately. Randomized trials
addressing this issue are currently in progress. If
anticoagulant therapy is given in acute stroke it is best
initiated gradually over several days with warfarin

— Reducing high blood pressure reduces the risk of subsequent
vascular events; however, hypotensive treatment in acute
stroke should be delayed for a few days, and a diastolic
blood pressure (phase 5) of up to 120 mmHg is acceptable
provided there are no grade 3 or 4 fundal signs or evidence
of left ventricular strain. Urgent treatment of higher blood
pressures should not be too vigorous, normalizing over days
rather than hours. Over-enthusiastic treatment of raised
blood pressure carries the risk of inducing hypotension and
reduced blood flow to the brain, which may result in further
ischaemia.

Increased blood pressure often occurs as a result of the
stroke, with diastolic blood pressures of 110–120 mmHg
being recorded especially during the first 48 hours after the
stroke. These raised blood pressures usually settle
spontaneously.

The older the patient the more cautious one should be
about any attempts to lower blood pressure.

In the first instance a thiazide diuretic should be tried to
reduce the diastolic blood pressure to about 100–110 mmHg;
if this alone is not effective a low dose of a beta-adrenergic
blocking drug may be added. The early morning diastolic
blood pressure should not be lowered much below
110 mmHg. One should watch vigorously for symptoms of
orthostatic hypotension.

In patients with subarachnoid haemorrhage raised blood pressure should
not be lowered before surgery; monitoring of fluid balance is also
extremely important, since both dehydration and reduction of blood
pressure carry a particular risk of inducing ischaemic infarction in these
patients. Blood pressure should only be lowered if it remains high after
surgery.

Prognosis

10–20% of stroke patients die within one month of a first stroke. The risk of recurrent stroke is about 4–5% per year. Early deaths are more likely to be due to the stroke (within 1 week) and to pulmonary embolism (2nd to 4th week), later deaths to bronchopneumonia (2nd and 3rd month) and to cardiac disease, mainly myocardial infarction (more than 3 months). Of the survivors of stroke about 15% return to normal or near normal function, though one must bear in mind that many elderly patients are already disabled due to conditions other than stroke.

The likelihood of death is increased by
— Prolonged coma
— Persistent conjugate deviation of the eyes
— Coexistent other illness (pulmonary embolus, bronchopneumonia, myocardial infarction)

BIBLIOGRAPHY

Anonymous 1985 Management of stroke. Drug and Therapeutics Bulletin 23: 9–12

Coakley D 1981 Stroke and other neurological emergencies in old age. In: Coakley D (ed) Acute geriatric medicine. Croom Helm, London, ch 3, pp 59–80

Consensus Conference 1988 Treatment of stroke. British Medical Journal 297: 126–128

ESPS Group 1987 The European Stroke Prevention Study (ESPS): Principal end-points. Lancet 2: 1351–1354

McCarthy S T, Turner J 1986 Low dose subcutaneous heparin in the prevention of deep vein thrombosis and pulmonary emboli following acute stroke. Age and Ageing 15: 84–88

Treseder A S, Sastry B S D, Thomas T P L, Yates M A, Pathy M S J 1986 Atrial fibrillation and stroke in elderly hospitalized patients. Age and Ageing 15: 89–92

Viitanen M, Winblad B, Asplund K 1987 Autopsy-verified causes of death after stroke. Acta Medica Scandinavica 222: 401–408

Wade D T, Langton Hewer R L 1983 Why admit stroke patients to hospital? Lancet 1: 807–809

Warlow C P 1987 Cerebrovascular disease. In Weatherall D J, Ledingham J G G, Warrel D A (eds) Oxford textbook of medicine. Oxford University Press, Oxford

2. STROKE REHABILITATION

The overall plan of rehabilitation of the patient embraces treatment of the organic disorder and the restoration of his capacity for biological adaptation to his environment. The success of rehabilitation will be judged on the degree of recovery of the physical, psychological and social functions.

Thus, it is convenient to make a triple functional assessment, both from the point of view of the understanding of the illness and for the formulation of the plan of rehabilitation.

Functional assessment

Physical assessment
Physical rehabilitation has as its aim the recovery of the maximum degree of physical function, and this may in many instances of stroke be incomplete. With medical treatment and with the restoration of function by physiotherapy, opportunities must be provided for the patient to become self-sufficient. This may require bed exercises, ward exercises, the use of special aids, prostheses, occupational therapy and devices to help in domestic tasks.

It is important to realize that rehabilitation is a process in which the patient engages, and what the patient achieves is done by him and not to him.

Severe limitations of physical capacity remaining after rehabilitation may necessitate a radical change in the physical and social environment. In other cases, where the residual disability is less serious, it may be possible for the patient to maintain a relatively independent existence by the provision of special appliances or mechanical aids in the home.

Psychological assessment
Personal reactions to illness include the following:

Loss of self-confidence
In the case of stroke, the illness and disability shatter the patient's self-confidence. The patient may come to realize that he may never again feel his former self.

Loss of independence
All illness brings with it some degree of dependency. In the acute stage of stroke this is likely to be maximal and the patient should receive all the attention and help possible. In the long term, the stroke may result in partial dependency.

Depression, loneliness and mental disturbances
Depression is a common feature in stroke patients. In addition, the physical incapacity caused by the stroke often restricts the patient's activities and prevents him from engaging in social relationships in the outside world, thus increasing his sense of loneliness and the chance of depression. Moreover, allowances must be made for the mental and behavioural disturbances which result from brain damage. Patience and understanding are therefore necessary; it must be realized that the apparent 'lack of initiative', 'poor cooperation' and 'unsuitable temperament' which stroke patients may exhibit may well be the results of the brain lesion. In addition, brain damage may result in personality deterioration, memory defects, confusion, mental disorientation and diminution in powers of concentration.

Social and environmental assessment
A study of an elderly person's domestic and family life is necessary to see how he was managing his everyday life before the stroke. The domestic care of the patient may throw a tremendous strain on others. It is thus necessary to assess the severity of the burden imposed by the patient, the effect this is having on the relatives, and also the family spirit in meeting their responsibilities. The general practitioner has usually made these assessments and is naturally often called upon to give advice both to the hospital multidisciplinary team and to the patient and his relatives.

 — In the case of an elderly stroke patient living alone it is particularly important to assess the performance of activities of daily living such as washing, dressing, cooking and shopping. The extent of the help given by neighbours or relatives should be ascertained as part of the multidisciplinary care plan

Assessment of deficits caused by the stroke

It is the disability caused by the stroke that is most important to the patient and his carers. For most patients the stay in hospital s a short prelude to a lifelong disability.

Paralysis
The missing functions in all stroke patients with paralysis consist of

1. Loss of the normal postural reflex mechanism on the affected side, and therefore, inability to initiate movement on this side

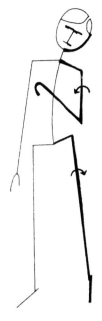

(a) TYPICAL SPASTICITY PATTERN

Retraction of shoulder with depression and internal rotation.

Forearm flexion.

Finger flexion with adduction.

Retraction of pelvis with external rotation of the leg.

Hip, knee and ankle extension with inversion and plantar flexion of the ankle

(b) ANTI-SPASTICITY OR RECOVERY PATTERN

Protraction of shoulder with external rotation.

Forearm extension.

Finger extension with abduction.

Protraction of pelvis with internal rotation of the leg.

Hip, knee and ankle flexion.

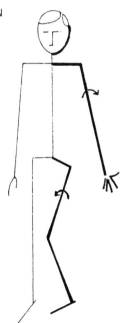

Fig. 2.1 Spasticity and anti-spasticity patterns. From Johnstone 1978.

2. Developing hypertonicity (spasticity) in the anti-gravity muscles (i.e. leg extensors, arm flexors)
3. Usually some degree of sensory disturbance which inhibits movement
4. As a consequence, there is a complete loss of free selection of precision movements on the affected side

The postural tone of the two sides is different

— At first, the patient's affected side is flaccid; he seems too weak to move his arm or leg; this may last for a few days up to a few weeks; in a few cases, flaccidity may persist indefinitely; flaccidity affects the arm more and for longer periods than the leg
— Spasticity then develops
— The typical spasticity pattern (Fig. 2.1a) is
— Arm
  • Retraction of the affected shoulder with depression and internal rotation
  • Forearm flexion, usually accompanied by pronation
  • Finger flexion with adduction
— Leg
  • Retraction of the pelvis with external rotation of the leg
  • Hip, knee and ankle extension with inversion and plantar flexion of the ankle
— Trunk
  • Lateral flexion of the trunk to the affected side

If spasticity becomes severe, it can result in contractures. It always interferes with the patient's ability to move later on. Correct positioning and handling of the stroke patient will prevent the abnormal postural patterns from becoming established.

— Positioning of the stroke patient consists of using the anti-spasm (or recovery) pattern at all times, from the day of onset of the stroke

The anti-spasticity or recovery pattern (Fig. 2.1b) is

— Arm
  • Protraction of the shoulder with external rotation
  • Forearm extension with supination
  • Finger extension with abduction
— Leg
  • Protraction of the pelvis with internal rotation of the leg
  • Hip, knee and ankle flexion
— Trunk
  • Elongation of the trunk on the affected side

A flaccid shoulder joint may be overstretched if excessive force is used while turning the patient.

— Shoulder care in the early days includes the prevention of a painful shoulder by support of the paralysed arm and early exercises, for example as illustrated in Figures 2.2–2.4

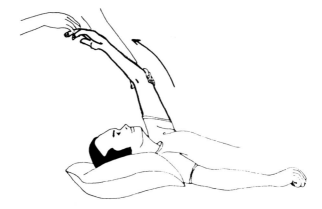

Fig. 2.2 Arm elevation with outward rotation. From Johnstone 1978.

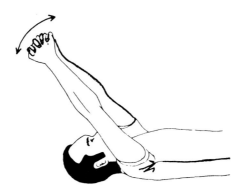

Fig. 2.3 Arm elevation: self-care. From Johnstone 1978.

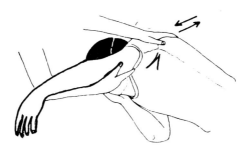

Fig. 2.4 Scapula movements. From Johnstone 1978.

— While maintaining protraction of the shoulder with external rotation, full elevation of the arm must be an early exercise. It will be practised in supine lying with a pillow placed under the hip to prevent retraction or a dropping backwards of the pelvis with external rotation of the leg. The pillow holds the hip in protraction and the knee is flexed with internal rotation of the hip. Supporting pillows may be placed under the thigh. Scapula movements must also be given with the patient lying on his sound side (Fig. 2.4)
— Frozen shoulder in upper limb paralysis is a long-term complication of stroke

Management

— Physiotherapy begins at an early stage, even if the patient is unconscious, since putting a patient through a passive range of movements may prevent contractures
— By being aware of the importance of early positioning of the stroke patient all staff can help to improve the patient's prospects of recovering optimal mobility.

Skeletal muscle relaxants

If necessary, skeletal muscle relaxants can be prescribed but only in patients with severe spasticity which hinders rehabilitation.

— Indications for prescribing are: spasticity and flexor/extensor spasms
— General rules
  • Dose should be increased slowly to prevent hypotonia and sedation
  • Drug withdrawal should be gradual

Preparations

1. *Baclofen*
   — Initially 5 mg tds, increasing by 5 mg added to each dose every 3–4 days, if necessary, to 20 mg qds
     • Disadvantages
       – Side effects: nausea, vomiting, diarrhoea; sedation, confusion; muscle hypotonia, fatigue; may aggravate depression
     • Contraindications
       – Should not be given to patients liable to epilepsy
     • Caution: higher risk of unwanted effects in
       – Patients with: peptic ulceration, cerebrovascular disease, hypotension, renal insufficiency, psychiatric disturbances
       – Elderly patients
     In these patients the dose should be increased very cautiously.

Note: Also use with caution in patients in whom spasticity is used to maintain posture or increase function

    2. *Diazepam*
- Initially 5 mg, increasing by 5 mg every third day until spasticity is relieved
  - Disadvantages
    - Lack of effect in severe spasticity
    - Side effects: sedation, confusion; fatigue

    3. *Dantrolene*
- Initially 25 mg
- Increase gradually over about 7 weeks to a maximum of 100 mg qds
- Usual dose is 75 mg tds
- If there is no response after 45 days: stop treatment
  - Disadvantages
    - High incidence of side effects: drowsiness, dizziness; weakness, malaise, fatigue; diarrhoea; hepatotoxicity in doses over 400 mg/day for over 60 days (monitor liver functions)
  - Contraindication
    - Pre-existing liver disease
  - Caution
    - Use with caution in patients with impaired pulmonary or cardiac function
    - In large doses it can weaken the muscles of the limbs and trunk

Visual/sensory inattention

These add considerably to the patient's difficulties and are a serious handicap to effective treatment and recovery. Sensory inattention may result in denial of the affected side. In addition, loss of spatial awareness and loss of position sense may be present. Where there is a sensory deficit sensory input must be stepped up.

Use

- Hearing: commands given must be short, dynamic and delivered from the correct place to gain a response
  - Example: if movement is to be to the right the member of staff will stand on the right
- Vision: used as above; the patient may be asked to watch his hand or foot when movement is required distal to proximal; a mirror may be useful
- Touch: plays a big part in sensory re-education; includes the use of light and deep pressure

Approaching the patient on the affected side and giving stimuli on the affected side are cornerstones of successful rehabilitation.

Homonymous hemianopia

Blindness in one half of the visual field of one or both eyes. Owing to this visual loss the patient, when learning to walk, may collide with objects on the affected side. Improvement can be expected and the patient who is aware of the deficit can be taught to rotate his head to compensate for the hopefully temporary disability. The patient should be encouraged to rotate across the affected side and, again, stimuli should be given on the affected side, such as placing the locker on the affected side.

Dysphagia

In patients with a pseudobulbar palsy or a brain stem stroke, dysphagia may make it necessary to establish IV or nasogastric feeding. Initial nutritional management with nasogastric feeding is often inappropriate because many of these patients have poor stomach emptying and there is a risk of regurgitation and aspiration into the lungs. Therefore, initial fluid replacement should be given IV on the paralysed side. If the swallowing reflexes have not returned after about 10 days, nasogastric feeding may be inevitable.

— Swallowing is often impaired in the early days after a stroke
— Semi-solids are preferable to solids or liquids in order to minimize the risk of aspiration. This aspect of care should be discussed with relatives if the patient goes home quite soon after the stroke

Aphasia/dysphasia

This occurs in left-sided lesions in right-handed individuals. The disturbance may be

1. Expressive (motor) aphasia consisting of an inability to express ideas through written or spoken language
2. Receptive (sensor) aphasia or impairment of understanding of oral or graphic symbols
3. Mixed aphasia, where there is disturbance in both expression and reception of language

Speech recovers better in patients with brain injury from trauma than in those with strokes. Aphasia/dysphasia is not only a handicap in itself, but also makes the work of the physiotherapist, occupational therapist and relatives harder. A speech therapist should assess the patients with communicative difficulty, even if they do not have the time to treat them, to determine at what level the patient is functioning. The prognosis is better in the expressive (motor) variety than in the receptive (sensor) variety. Speech therapy can be given at home depending on local resources. Relatives can be involved in it.

Failure to understand instructions

Apart from the speech problems that may be present, the lack of visual, sensory and proprioceptive pathways may leave the patient confused and unable to carry out instructions. In addition, the acute illness that may be associated with the stroke may cause a considerable degree of confusion in an elderly patient (for example: atrial fibrillation not yet controlled; basal pneumonia due to lack of inflation of the lung basis on the affected side, or due to aspiration; uncontrolled diabetes). There may be a mild premorbid dementia: try and check with relatives whether memory has been impaired prior to the stroke, and whether there is any evidence of abnormal behaviour or disorientation prior to the stroke (see also Ch. 5).

Apraxia

This consists of an inability to carry out purposed movements in the absence of severe paralysis, ataxia or sensory loss. There is usually difficulty in performing skilled actions with the hands, but a condition of ambulatory apraxia may occur.

Depression

Depression is common both in the patient and the relatives; it may interfere with rehabilitation and feeding; it may occur or worsen after discharge from hospital, especially if preparation for discharge has been inadequate; counselling of the patient and the relatives, referral to stroke groups and/or stroke support groups, access to information such as the Chest, Heart and Stroke Association booklet, support for and relief of the main carer will help to prevent depression; antidepressant therapy may help if the depression dominates the patient's life. (see also Ch. 6). Anxiety and personality changes may also occur in patients who have suffered a stroke.

Urinary incontinence

— This commonly develops as a result of loss of cortical inhibition (see also Ch. 26). The uninhibited neurogenic bladder has hypertonic and hyperexcitable musculature. In some cases there is difficulty in micturition, with retention of urine; this may lead to 'overflow' incontinence
— In the acute stage of stroke condom drainage is most suitable for incontinent men, unless there is urine retention, in which case catheterization is necessary. An indwelling catheter is usually necessary for incontinent women. Catheters should be removed and bowel and bladder training commenced as early as possible
— In later stages, troublesome constipation can hinder bladder emptying
— In addition, the immobility caused by the stroke may contribute to the persistence of urinary incontinence
— Also, urinary tract infection is a common general complication of stroke

Barriers to rehabilitation and functional recovery

— Hemianaesthesia
  • Denial of affected side (visual/sensory inattention)
  • Loss of spatial awareness
  • Loss of position sense

— Hemianopia
— Presence of brain failure
— Depression/anxiety/personality changes
— Dysphasia (sensory worse than motor)
— Thalamic syndrome

In general, an early assessment of the patient's disabilities and early implementation of a multidisciplinary care plan are corner-stones of successful rehabilitation of stroke patients. A hospitalized stroke patient should not be discharged home until adequate preparations have been made for both the patient and the carer. For some patients, a home assessment together with the physiotherapist or occupational therapist may be required prior to discharge from hospital. After discharge the general practitioner should be asked to be the key person to coordinate further rehabilitation and reassess the patient regularly.

BIBLIOGRAPHY

Allen C M C 1984 Predicting recovery after acute stroke. British Journal of Hospital Medicine 31: 428–434
Bobath B 1978 Adult hemiplegia: Evaluation and treatment. Heinemann, London
Exton-Smith A N (ed) 1955 Rehabilitation: The patient with hemiplegia. In: Medical problems of old age. Wright, Bristol. ch 7, pp 75–86
Johnstone M 1978 Restoration of motor function in the stroke patient. Churchill Livingstone, Edinburgh

3 TRANSIENT ISCHAEMIC ATTACKS

Definition (WHO 1971)

The sudden occurrence of usually repeated episodes of sensory or motor impairment, caused by temporary inadequacy of blood flow to a localized area of the brain and disappearing completely within 24 hours. Most TIAs last less than 1 hour.

Epidemiology

In the UK, approximately 25 000 people per year experience their first TIA. The incidence increases rapidly with age; the annual age-adjusted incidence for the UK is 0.5 TIA/1000.

Precipitating factors

The basic pathology, in particular in the carotid region, is thought to be atheroma with microemboli arising from the atheromatous plaque.

Patients must be evaluated for evidence of
  — Arterial disease
  — Cardiac disease, including cardiac dysrhythmia and heart block
  — Blood disorders: anaemia, polycythaemia, thrombocythaemia
  — Changes in serum glucose level
  — Hyperlipaemia
  — Rare disorders, such as leukaemia, thrombotic thrombocytopenic purpura, 'hyperviscosity' syndromes (e.g. myeloma), sickle-cell disease

Clinical picture

Symptoms and/or signs vary depending on the part of the brain affected. Loss of consciousness may occur, but is a rare phenomenon. TIAs may occur either in the carotid region or in the vertebrobasilar region. They are important warning signs of impending stroke and occur in 10–20% of all patients who develop a stroke. The greatest risk of developing a stroke is possibly within the first year.

Presenting features

TIAs in the carotid region

These are more serious and symptoms include
- — Amaurosis fugax (transient monocular loss of vision)
- — Language disturbance (dominant hemisphere): dysphasia, transient word blindness
- — Dysarthria
- — Visuospatial disorientation (non-dominant hemisphere)
- — Monoparesis/hemiparesis/facial hemiparesis
- — Hemiparaesthesia/hemianaesthesia

Symptoms are usually of the same type in each attack.

TIAs in the vertebrobasilar region

They may present with
- — Falls/ataxia
- — Nystagmus
- — Vertigo
- — Nausea and vomiting
- — Episodes of hypotension
- — Impairment of thermoregulation

If both occipital cortices are involved
- — Cortical blindness may occur

If one occipital cortex is involved
- — Homonymous hemianopia with macular sparing may occur

If the cranial nerve nuclei are involved, there may be
- — Dysphagia
- — Dysarthria
- — Diplopia
- — Hemiparesis or tetraparesis
- — Hemianaesthesia or bilateral sensory loss
- — Perioral paraesthesia
- — Unilateral facial sensory loss with contralateral motor and/or sensory disturbance in the limbs

Differential diagnosis

Conditions to be considered
- — Migraine
- — Epilepsy
- — Psychogenic
- — Hypoglycaemia
- — Arteriovenous malformations
- — Subdural haematoma
- — Intracerebral haemorrhage
- — Tumour

CT scan of the brain is required to exclude the latter four conditions.

Assessment

Patients presenting with a TIA should be screened for evidence of any of the precipitating factors mentioned above.

Investigations
- ESR
- Full blood count
- Serum glucose level
- Urea and electrolytes
- Serum creatinine level
- Hepatic function
- Urine examination
- Chest X-ray (CXR)
- Electrocardiogram (ECG)
- 24-hour electrocardiographic monitoring (on indication)
- Echocardiography (on indication)

Management

Surgical approach
- In cases of carotid territory TIAs check the patient for carotid stenosis, which may reveal itself by a bruit in the neck or by inequality of internal carotid pulsation in the neck
- If either is found, or if the patient's history is strongly indicative for a carotid territory TIA, the patient ought to be referred to a vascular surgeon.

Non-invasive techniques used in assessing carotid flow
- Doppler recording
- Ophthalmodynamometry
- Facial thermometry

Their value lies in preliminary screening; the nature of the obstruction can only be defined by
- A carotid angiogram: this should only be carried out in patients who are considered fit for surgery. The most common site of atheroma is the origin of the internal carotid artery; this is the only site which is accessible to surgery and carotid endarterectomy. If a significant isolated carotid stenosis is found, carotid endarterectomy could perhaps achieve cessation of attacks and prevent a completed stroke; this issue is currently being addressed in both a European and Northern American clinical trial. Carotid endarterectomy is usually not done in patients over 70 years old, because the operation has a high morbidity and high mortality in this age group
- When multiple sites of atherosclerotic disease are found on

angiography or when the patient is not fit for surgery, medical treatment must be considered (see later).

In vertebrobasilar territory TIAs the precise aetiology is not known, though microemboli arising from atheromatous plaque in the vertebrobasilar tree are thought to be a causal factor. There is no clear correlation with vascular stenosis as is the case in carotid territory TIAs. Thus, there is no surgical approach and the first line of treatment is medical.

Medical treatment

Anticoagulant therapy
This does not appear to alter survival after the onset of TIAs and is now only indicated in the following groups of patients
1. Patients with a TIA who have rheumatic cardiac valve disease
2. Patients with a TIA who suffered a recent myocardial infarction (short-term cover)
3. A European trial is addressing the issue of no treatment, or treatment with anticoagulant therapy or aspirin (acetylsalicylic acid) for patients with TIA and atrial fibrillation in the absence of other cardiac abnormalities

Aspirin
In all other patients aspirin is the treatment of choice: 300 mg daily lifelong unless contraindications occur. If indigestion occurs, combination with an antacid should be considered.

Note: The addition of dipyridamole to aspirin confers no advantage.

Contraindications for anticoagulant therapy
— Hypertension
— Hypertensive or diabetic retinopathy
— (Previous) haemorrhage or predisposition to haemorrhage, for example: hiatus hernia, peptic ulcer, thrombocytopenia
— Serious renal failure
— Serious parenchymatous liver disease
— Poor compliance

Contraindications for aspirin
— Peptic ulcer
— (Previous) haemorrhage in the gastrointestinal tract
— Allergy to acetylsalicylic acid
— Poor compliance

Caution: Aspirin is known to enhance the effect of insulin and of oral hypoglycaemic drugs, so hypoglycaemica could be induced; it is also known to enhance the effect of methotrexate, increasing the chance of occurrence of a serious blood disorder.

BIBLIOGRAPHY

Barnett H J M 1979 The pathophysiology of transient cerebral ischaemic attacks. Medical Clinics of North America 63: 649–679

Canadian Co-operative Study Group 1978 A randomised trial of aspirin and sulfinpyrazone in threatened stroke. New England Journal of Medicine 299: 53–59

Marshall J 1971 Angiography in the investigation of ischaemic episodes in territory of the internal carotid artery. Lancet 1: 719–721

Millikan C H, McDowell F H 1978 Treatment of transient ischaemic attacks. Stroke 9: 299–308

Sandok B A, Furlan A J, Whisnant J P, Sundt T M 1978 Guidelines for the management of transient ischaemic attacks. Mayo Clinic Proceedings 53: 665–674

Winslow C M, Solomon D H, Chassin M R et al 1988 The appropriateness of carotid endarterectomy. New England Journal of Medicine 318: 721–727

Whisnant J P, Matsumoto N, Elveback L R 1973 The effect of anticoagulation therapy on the prognosis of patients with transient cerebral ischaemic attacks in a community, Rochester, Minnesota, 1955 through 1969. Mayo Clinic Proceedings 48: 844–848

Yeung Laiwah A C 1983 Management of transient cerebral ischaemic attacks by hospital doctors in Scotland. Journal of the Royal College of Physicians of London 17: 173–177

4. PARKINSON'S DISEASE

Parkinson's disease (idiopathic parkinsonism, paralysis agitans) was first described by James Parkinson in 1817 in 'An Essay on the Shaking Palsy'. It is a clinical syndrome characterized by three cardinal features: hypokinesia, tremor and rigidity. In Parkinson's disease the aetiology is unknown and hence it is often referred to as idiopathic parkinsonism. Some patients develop parkinsonism as a result of infections (encephalitis lethargica, syphilitic mesencephalitis, tuberculoma), drugs (phenothiazines, butyrophenones, rauwolfia alkaloids, tetrabenazine), boxing, or carbon monoxide poisoning. Secondary parkinsonism occurs in a few syndromes such as the Shy–Drager syndrome and progressive supranuclear palsy. Idiopathic parkinsonism must also be differentiated from hyperkinetic syndromes such as senile chorea, Huntington's chorea, dyskinesias and senile dystonia.

The term 'arteriosclerotic parkinsonism' has been used to describe the akinesia of multi-infarct cerebral disorder and is no longer considered a true entity, since there is no evidence of vascular disease in the basal ganglia.

Pathology

All forms of parkinsonism are characterized by dopamine deficiency in the corpus striatum in the basal ganglia. This results in an imbalance of dopamine and acetylcholine neurotransmitters in the brain. In idiopathic parkinsonism the main pathological findings are loss of pigmentation in the substantia nigra and, to a lesser extent, in the locus coeruleus pontis and dorsal nucleus of the vagus, and the presence of Lewy bodies and other types of intraneuronal inclusion bodies (i.e. eosinophilic structures, measuring approximately 20 μm in diameter) in many diencephalic and brain stem nuclei, in the lateral and posterior horns of the spinal cord and in the ganglia of the sympathetic chain. Idiopathic parkinsonism is thought to arise from degeneration of the dopaminergic nigrostriatal pathways. Patients with postencephalitic parkinsonism also show loss of pigmentation in the substantia nigra, but the most characteristic finding is the severe neurofibrillary degeneration in substantia nigra, putamen, thalamus, hypothalamus and other structures; Lewy bodies are not found in postencephalitic parkinsonism.

Epidemiology

The prevalence of idiopathic parkinsonism in Europe and North America is approximately 2000 per 100 000 above 70 years of age; under 50 years of age the prevalence is only 8 per 100 000. Both sexes are affected approximately equally.

Postencephalitic parkinsonism was a complication of encephalitis lethargica or sleepy sickness, of which there were several epidemics in the years following 1919. Of all patients with postencephalitic parkinsonism, 80% developed their symptoms within 10 years of the infection. During the 1920s, approximately 65% of cases of parkinsonism were of the postencephalitic type. In the 1930s, the figure was still 50%. Today postencephalitic parkinsonism is less significant, as few new cases occur.

Clinical features

Essential to the diagnosis of idiopathic parkinsonism is the presence of hypokinesia and rigidity; resting tremor completes the triad, but its presence is not essential to the diagnosis.

Hypokinesia

The most disabling component of the disease; the term is used to describe slowness in the initiation and execution of voluntary motor acts and a general poverty of automatic and associated movements. Little is known about the physiological basis of this phenomenon, which probably accounts, in part at least, for many parkinsonian symptoms and signs, such as

— Reduced blinking
— Impaired ocular divergence
— Mask-like facies
— Monotonous speech (amounting at times to virtual anarthria)
— Micrographia
— Reduced swinging of the arms while walking

In the elderly the hypokinesia tends to be bilateral and symmetrical from onset. In some patients the hypokinesia dominates the clinical picture, rendering the patient housebound or even chairbound.

Rigidity

Common in all types of parkinsonism; it may be unilateral, though in the elderly it tends to be bilateral and symmetrical from onset; it appears early in the musculature of the neck, contributing to the characteristic 'flexed posture'. It is detected clinically by resistance to passive movement. 'Cogwheel rigidity' is not just parkinsonian rigidity complicated by parkinsonian tremor, for it may occur in the absence of resting tremor and its frequency is often higher (6–12 cycles/second compared to 4–8 cycles/second for the tremor). The 'flexed posture' contributes to the phenomena of anteropulsion and festinant (hurrying) gait.

Tremor

The presenting complaint in over 65% of patients with idiopathic parkinsonism. It usually affects distal muscles, such as those of the hand, forearm or foot. The tremor is characteristically present at rest and decreases on movement; it is made worse by nervousness, excitement or fatigue.

It may produce flexion–extension movements of the fingers or pronation–supination movements of the forearm. Occasionally the foot alone may be involved, or the jaw or tongue may be affected. The tremor rate varies from 4 to 8 cycles/second.

Other symptoms

Mental disturbances

1. Depression is common, especially in patients with insight into the decline of their faculties.
2. Inertia is often present; the patient may recognize it, but seems unable to do anything about it.
3. Chronic brain failure of varying degrees has been associated with parkinsonism; this association was described prior to the levodopa era and is more obvious with longer survival due to levodopa therapy. Debate continues about the nature of parkinsonian dementia and it is thought to be multifactorial in origin.

Drooling of saliva

In patients with advanced parkinsonism this is primarily caused by mechanical factors, and there is no evidence that hypersecretion occurs.

Dysphagia

Common in patients with parkinsonism; radiological studies may show a delay in the initiation of swallowing. Aspiration may occur.

Heartburn

Common, at least 25% of patients with parkinsonism have a hiatus hernia and gastro-oesophageal reflux.

Weight loss

Common: 75% of patients with parkinsonism are below their optimal weight.

Postural disorders

Commonly occur in patients with parkinsonism. Patients may be unable to stand unaided and tend to fall without the usual defensive reactions. Unexpected falls may be the presenting feature of parkinsonism. In late-onset parkinsonism the disorder of posture and balance occurs earlier in the course of the disease and tends to dominate the clinical picture to a greater degree than in younger patients.

Autonomic dysfunction

May occur due to the disease and is a common phenomenon in elderly parkinsonian patients; symptoms may include

— Postural hypotension

— Defective bladder control
— Distressing constipation, sometimes leading to megacolon and large bowel obstruction, and even to unnecessary laparotomies

Differential diagnosis

In the elderly, idiopathic parkinsonism must be differentiated mainly from essential tremor, postencephalitic parkinsonism and drug-induced parkinsonism.

Essential tremor
This is an action tremor and disappears with complete relaxation. It affects the hands much more frequently than parkinsonian tremor and almost always spares the legs. In addition, only essential tremor involves the jaw, face and voice. Patients with essential tremor do not have rigidity.

Postencephalitic parkinsonism
Rare: characterized by a past history of encephalitis, onset early in life, non-progression or very slow progression, and by a number of special features such as tics, oculogyric spasms and marked skeletal deformities (scoliosis, wrist and hand deformities).

Drug-induced parkinsonism
Most common in elderly subjects. The predilection of the elderly to develop drug-induced parkinsonism generally reflects the high incidence of the disease in the over-70 age group and the progressive loss of substantia nigra cells with normal ageing. Such nigral cell loss remains compensated without clinical parkinsonism until the remaining cells are depleted by drugs such as reserpine and tetrabenazine, or postsynaptic receptor block occurs with phenothiazines or butyrophenones. Drug-induced parkinsonism of short duration is usually reversible.

Management

Treatment of parkinsonism consists of drugs, physiotherapy, occupational therapy and supportive care.

Drugs
Levodopa
The drug of choice for the treatment of parkinsonism in old age. It was introduced in the latter part of the 1960s and revolutionized the treatment of parkinsonism. Treatment is based on the concept that levodopa, the amino acid precursor of dopamine, can compensate for the deficiency of striatal dopamine by being converted to dopamine in the remaining nigral neurons. This, in turn, provides for stimulation of the denervated postsynaptic striatal dopamine receptors. Levodopa has a plasma half-life varying from 45 minutes to 1.5 hours. The main

excretory products are homovanillic acid and dihydroxyphenylacetic acid. Levodopa improves all the clinical features of parkinsonism. Additionally, life expectancy is virtually normalized in levodopa-treated patients with idiopathic parkinsonism. If a patient reports no improvement on levodopa therapy, the diagnosis of idiopathic parkinsonism should be reviewed. Effective treatment with levodopa is limited mainly by nausea and vomiting. For this reason preparations containing levodopa and a dopa-decarboxylase inhibitor are now widely used in geriatric practice. Dopa-decarboxylase inhibitors are carbidopa and benserazide. They inhibit the enzyme which is responsible for the conversion of levodopa to dopamine. They do not cross the blood–brain barrier, and so reduce the peripheral breakdown of levodopa to dopamine outside the central nervous system, allowing a higher concentration of levodopa to enter the central nervous system, where it is converted to dopamine at the site where it is needed — the striatum. By adding carbidopa or benserazide to levodopa the dose of levodopa can be reduced by 80% without plasma concentration falling, and certain adverse reactions of levodopa (such as emesis and cardiac arrhythmias) are reduced. No side effects have been described from carbidopa or benserazide.

The main side effects of levodopa are those arising within the central nervous system, such as dyskinesia (i.e. bizarre movements), confusion, hallucinations and delusions; it must be used very cautiously in an old person already mildly confused. It should not be used in conjunction with any psychotropic drugs which affect cerebral amine metabolism. Other side effects are restlessness and (orthostatic) hypotension (common), and cardiac arrhythmias, gout and hot flushes (rare).

Long-term problems are a loss of efficacy (i.e. a loss of response to levodopa treatment with progression of the disease) and fluctuations in motor performance such as 'end-of-dose' deterioration (i.e. a wearing off of the beneficial response to levodopa prior to the onset of benefit from the subsequent dose) and the 'on–off' phenomenon (i.e. extreme fluctuations between 'on' periods in which patients are relatively free from parkinsonian symptoms but may suffer disabling dyskinesias and 'off' periods in which patients lose their response to medication and may become severely rigid and akinetic).

Preparations
1. Sinemet-275: levodopa 250 mg and carbidopa 25 mg
2. Sinemet-110: levodopa 100 mg and carbidopa 10 mg
3. Sinemet Plus: levodopa 100 mg and carbidopa 25 mg
4. Madopar-250: levodopa 200 mg and benserazide 50 mg
5. Madopar-125: levodopa 100 mg and benserazide 25 mg
   — Start with Sinemet-110 twice a day
   — Increments should be made of one Sinemet-110 tablet at a time
   — Few elderly patients tolerate more than the equivalent of Sinemet-275 thrice daily

— General rule: small doses at frequent intervals are often better than larger doses at fixed intervals, because patients on higher doses tend to have 'on–off' effects. This problem may be alleviated by increasing the frequency of dosing but keeping the overall daily dose constant.

The effects of levodopa do not last forever. More than half of parkinsonian patients treated with levodopa for over 5 years begin to lose their beneficial response and develop adverse reactions. Therefore, other drugs have been tried.

Amantadine

This drug is less potent than levodopa; it improves all clinical features of parkinsonism; it is rapidly and completely absorbed from the gut; it has a long duration of action and is excreted unchanged in the urine. Its main indication is as additional treatment in patients who can tolerate only suboptimal doses of levodopa. One of its major drawbacks is the fading of effect after 4–8 weeks. It is relatively free from side effects in the doses usually prescribed, i.e. 100 mg once or twice daily. It can be given alone or in combination with levodopa. Side effects include: restlessness, dizziness, headache, confusion, hallucinations, nausea, cardiac arrhythmias and livedo reticularis. High doses can precipitate seizures and epilepsy is a relative contraindication. Cessation of therapy must be gradual since abrupt cessation can cause exacerbation of parkinsonism. Amantadine should be avoided in patients with severe renal impairment.

Bromocriptine

This drug is an artificial agonist of dopamine; it activates the dopamine receptors. Its pharmacokinetic and pharmacodynamic properties differ from levodopa. It is rapidly absorbed and metabolized; it is excreted mainly via the liver, only 6% is excreted via the kidneys. Plasma protein binding is 96%. It induces less dyskinesia than levodopa. The plasma half-life and therapeutic action are more prolonged, so there are fewer 'wearing off' reactions. It can be given alone or in combination with anticholinergic and/or other antiparkinsonian drugs. It is usually prescribed in patients with a reduced response to levodopa and in patients who have developed 'on–off' phenomenon while on levodopa therapy. Side effects are restlessness, confusion, hallucinations, nausea, orthostatic hypotension and painful legs.

A test dose of 1 mg should be given to check if the patient is sensitive to its hypotensive effect. Starting dose is 2.5 mg note, increasing slowly while the levodopa dosage is concurrently reduced. The usual daily dose is 10–15 mg, with a maximum daily dose of 30 mg.

Selegiline

This is a monoamine oxidase-B inhibitor used in severe parkinsonism together with levodopa. It has been suggested that by reducing the oxidation of dopamine this drug will conserve transmitter. It extends the period of response to each dose of levodopa and is used together with levodopa to reduce the 'end of dose' akinesia. The starting dose is 5 mg once a day, increasing to 10 mg once a day. The dose of levodopa usually has to be reduced by about 20% when patients are treated concomitantly with selegiline.

A side effect of selegiline is insomnia; it also increases the risk of levodopa-induced hallucinations.

Anticholinergic drugs
May be used to reduce tremor and rigidity but are less effective for the treatment of hypokinesia. Their use should be limited in the elderly because of a high incidence of side effects. Most frequently prescribed are benzhexol, orphenadrine and procyclidine. No advantage has been established for any one anticholinergic drug over another in the treatment of any one particular clinical feature of parkinsonism. Anticholinergic drugs are slowly increased to their maximum tolerated dose over a period of 1–2 months; the most commonly used anticholinergic drugs are:

	Initial dose	Maintenance dose
Benzhexol	1–2 mg od or bd	6–30 mg daily
Orphenadrine	50 mg od or bd	200–400 mg daily
Procyclidine	2.5–5 mg od	10–60 mg daily

Side effects are due to parasympathetic blockade and include pupillary dilatation, defective accommodation, dryness of mouth, tachycardia, constipation and retention of urine. The major CNS side effects are psychiatric symptoms, i.e. confusion, delusions and hallucinations.

Note
— Pupillary dilatation may precipitate an attack of acute glaucoma
— Dryness of mouth may induce difficulty in swallowing

Treatment of drug-induced parkinsonism
This condition is relieved by stopping the offending drug. It is usually reversible if it has been of short duration. Benztropine mesylate may be administered: starting dose 0.5 mg, maximum dose 2–4 mg. A parenteral preparation of 2 mg in 2 ml for IV or IM injection is available. Side effects are sedation, defective accommodation, dry mouth, nausea, exanthema, malaise.

BIBLIOGRAPHY

Hoehn M M 1986 Parkinson's disease: Progression and mortality. In Jahr M D, Bergmann K J (eds) Advances in Neurology. Raven Press, New York
Hoehn M M, Elton R L 1985 Low dosages of bromocriptine added to levodopa in Parkinson's disease. Neurology 35: 199–206

Nutt J G, Woodward W R, Hammerstad J P, Carter J H, Anderson J L 1984 The 'on–off' phenomenon in Parkinson's disease: Relation to levodopa absorption and transport. New England Journal of Medicine 1: 483–488

Olanow C W 1988 Current concepts in the treatment of Parkinson's disease. Journal for Drug Therapy and Research 13: 102–107

Rajput A H, Stern W, Laverty W H 1984 Chronic low dose levodopa therapy in Parkinson's disease. Neurology 34: 991–996

Rinne U K 1985 Combined bromocriptine–levodopa therapy early in Parkinson's disease. Neurology 35: 1196–1198

Rinne U K 1987 Early combination of bromocriptine and levodopa in the treatment of Parkinson's disease: A five year follow-up. Neurology 37: 826–828

5. DEMENTIA

Definition

Dementia is the global impairment of higher cortical functions, including
— Memory
— The capacity to solve the problems of day-to-day living
— The performance of learned perceptuomotor skills
— The correct use of social skills
— The control of emotional reactions
These impairments occur in the absence of gross clouding of
consciousness. The condition is often irreversible and progressive. This
definition was adopted by the Royal College of Physicians in its report
'Organic Mental Impairment in the Elderly' (1981). Nowadays, quite
often the term 'brain failure' is used, indicating that the patient has a
degree of failure of overall brain function.

Epidemiology

Dementia is a common disorder in modern societies because of the size
of their elderly populations. The prevalence of dementia rises with age:
5.0–7.1% of the over-65s have dementia, with prevalence rates rising
from about 2% at ages of 65–70 to around 20% at ages over 80. Similar
figures are reported from most countries in the Western world. Case
register studies of newly reported cases reveal an annual incidence of
1.5–5 per 1000 population over the age of 60. One of the demographic
facts of the ageing population in the UK is that up to the year 2000
there is likely to be a disproportionate increase (about 45%) in the
number of persons over the age of 85, the very group most likely to
contract dementia. This will impinge upon the practice of all branches of
the medical profession caring for elderly people and will present a great
challenge to medical practice.

Causes of dementia

Dementia is a functional, not a pathological term. The possible causes
are many, but most cases are associated with degenerative disease of the
CNS. In geriatric in-patients with dementia post-mortem studies have
attributed about 70% of cases to Alzheimer dementia, either alone
(50%) or in combination with multi-infarct dementia (20%). Another
15% of cases is attributed to multi-infarct dementia. The remainder
suffer from various other, less common but nevertheless important and

in some cases potentially reversible conditions (see list below). The brain is affected in different ways; the final expression is widespread neuronal failure and dementia.

Causes may be summarized as follows

— Common
  - Alzheimer dementia, including SDAT
  - Mixed Alzheimer dementia and multi-infarct dementia
  - Multi-infarct dementia
— Less common
  - Parkinson's disease
  - Huntington's chorea
  - Progressive supranuclear palsy
  - Progressive myoclonus epilepsy
  - Pick's disease
  - Creutzfeldt–Jakob disease
  - Wilson's disease
  - Infection (e.g. syphilis)
  - Hydrocephalus
  - Trauma
  - Metabolic and deficiency diseases

Conditions which may mimic dementia are acute confusional state (see Ch. 22) and depression (see Ch. 6).

ALZHEIMER DEMENTIA

Pathology

This is the most common type of dementia; it may occur in the senium (age >65) or in the pre-senium (age <65) but is rarely seen below the age of 50; the term 'Alzheimer's disease' used to be reserved for pre-senile cases, while 'senile dementia Alzheimer type' was used for patients aged over 65. Nowadays the term 'Alzheimer dementia' is most frequently used. However, there is reason to believe that a distinction may be made, i.e. between the rate of progression of the dementia in 'younger' and 'older' groups of patients. It is now thought that there are two forms, if not types, of Alzheimer dementia: one runs a severe course with a rapidly fatal outcome, and occurs in early-onset cases; the other has a less severe course with a less poor prognosis, and occurs in late-onset cases.

Alzheimer dementia cannot be diagnosed with certainty during life except by cortical biopsy. Therefore, most cases are diagnosed at post-mortem by the demonstration of senile plaques and neurofibrillary tangles throughout the cerebral cortex (see definitions below). In addition, granuvacuolar lesions and Hirano bodies — although confined to the hippocampus — are found more frequently than in normal old age (see Table 5.1).

Table 5.1

Alzheimer dementia	Normal ageing
Senile plaques and neurofibrillary tangles throughout cerebral cortex	Small numbers of senile plaques and neurofibrillary tangles — confined to hippocampus
Granulovacuolar degeneration and Hirano bodies in hippocampus frequent	Much less frequent
Severe cholinergic deficit present	Absent
Marked reduction of brain weight: brains from patients with Alzheimer dementia weigh ±10–15% less than those from age-matched non-demented persons	7–10% reduction of brain weight by ninth decade

— Senile plaques are neuritic plaques with a complex structure containing amyloid, degenerating synaptic terminals and neurites; in Alzheimer dementia they are found throughout the cerebral cortex
— Neurofibrillary tangles are abnormal neurons in which paired helical filaments accumulate in the neuronal soma and neurites; in Alzheimer dementia they are found in the hippocampus, amygdala, medial temporal lobes and frontal cortex
— Granuvacuolar degeneration means that intracellular vacuoles are present in hippocampal pyramidal neurons; each vacuole contains a single central 1–2-μm granule
— Hirano bodies are elongated eosinophilic structures in the hippocampus

The 'cholinergic hypothesis' of Alzheimer dementia can be described as follows: 'damage to the ascending cholinergic system is an important determinant of the functional deficits observed in Alzheimer dementia'. Acetylcholine, probably the main transmitter involved in higher neuronal activity, is reduced due to appreciable reductions in the activity of the enzyme choline acetyltransferase (ChAT, which synthesizes acetylcholine) in the cerebral cortex of patients with Alzheimer dementia. This cholinergic deficit, as assessed by ChAT activity, affects especially the hippocampus, amygdala and temporal cortex.

The earlier the age at death the more severe this cholinergic abnormality — in patients dying after the age of 80 the frontal lobe is unaffected (Fig. 5.1).

The reduction in ChAT activity correlates both with the density of cortical senile plaques and with the severity of dementia at the time of death, whereas there are no obvious correlations with other markers.

In addition to the cholinergic deficit, cortical concentrations of noradrenaline, gamma-aminobutyric acid (GABA) and somatostatin have been reported to be reduced in patients with Alzheimer dementia; again these deficits were found to be more obvious in early onset-cases.

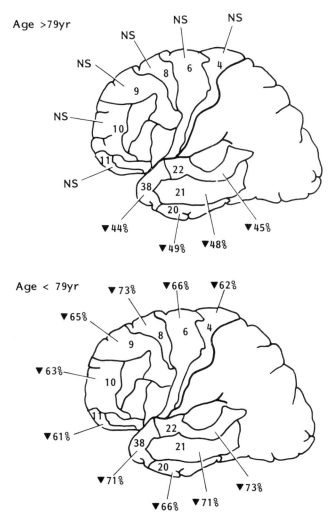

Fig. 5.1 ChAT activities in Alzheimer's disease. The figures are percentage reductions from age-matched control values. Reduced activity is seen in the temporal lobe at all ages but the frontal lobe deficit is confined to the younger group. Data derived from Rossor (1982).

Other neurotransmitter systems with projection to the cerebral cortex which have been reported to be abnormal in Alzheimer dementia are the serotoninergic and dopaminergic systems. However, the abnormalities in these systems have not been as clearly defined as the cholinergic and noradrenergic deficits.

In Alzheimer dementia the neuronal loss produces diffuse cerebral atrophy and enlargement of the ventricles and sulcal spaces. Studies have shown that in elderly subjects increasing age is associated with increasing brain atrophy; during human life maximum brain weight (1374 g) is reached at age 20; thereafter, there is a gradual decrease of brain weight so that by the ninth decade 7–10% of brain weight has been lost. In Alzheimer dementia brain weight is much more reduced, i.e. from 1200–1350 g to around 1000 g.

Clinical features

The impairment of memory and cognitive functions characteristic of Alzheimer dementia may not at first be apparent. This may be due to the fact that the degree of change is too subtle to be revealed by psychological assessment in the absence of pre-morbid quantitative estimations of functioning.

In the early stages the patient may deny memory impairment due to anxiety about its implications; alternatively, the patient may not recognize the loss of memory and cognitive functions due to concomitant impairment of judgement and insight. Thompson has stated that 'dementia is a latent condition, often detectable only by challenge'. Indeed, in many patients the diagnosis of dementia is not made until some other condition precipitates admission to hospital. Another early change is lack of initiative, which may lead to physical complaints such as 'tiredness' and hence to an initial consultation with a physician rather than a psychiatrist. As the dementia progresses, behavioural and personality changes may occur, with manifestations of irritability, aggressiveness, anger, restlessness, decline in moral standards, and the indulgence in antisocial acts. Paranoid delusions may occur, but one of the most common symptoms is depression. Since depression may affect the patient's performance on psychometric testing, it may be difficult to make the distinction between depression and dementia.

The later stages of Alzheimer dementia are associated with a variety of neurological changes, including

— Primitive reflexes, such as sucking and pouting reflexes, palmomental reflex, tonic grasp reflex (which occurs in association with a tonic foot response)
— Speech disorders: often loss of abstract thought results in signs of concrete thinking in the patient's speech; the patient may talk excessively and incoherently; dysphasia (sensory or motor) is always present to a variable degree; in the end stage echolalia or muteness may occur
— Dyspraxia: difficulty in putting movements together
— Spatial, visual and object agnosia
— Gait and postural disturbances such as the 'marche à petits pas', which is caused by motor apraxia and in which the person has a flexed stance with a slightly widened base and advances with slow, small steps; the flexion attitude of the elderly is present to a much greater degree in elderly demented patients because of an overall increase in tone (this can be differentiated from Parkinson's disease because of the lack of cogwheel rigidity and the lack of dyskinesia);

the overall increase in tone may result in flexion
contractures of arms and legs which may render the patient
immobile
— Focal weaknesses
— Convulsions
— Urinary and faecal incontinence occur due to deteriorating
cortical control of bladder and bowel

Prognosis
Until quite recently, the entire course of the average case of Alzheimer
dementia was thought to last 2–5 years; this was probably partly due to
late diagnosis; nowadays, the survival of the typical case of Alzheimer
dementia is thought to be nearer 10 years.

MULTI-INFARCT DEMENTIA

Pathology
This is considered to be due to the occurrence of multiple infarcts; the
condition is associated with cerebrovascular disease. The brain usually
shows unevenly distributed disintegration of cerebral tissue, often but not
always with evidence of large or microscopic infarcts. It is their presence
which has led to the use of the term 'multi-infarct dementia', now
preferred to the use of the term 'arteriosclerotic dementia'. Dementia
seldom occurs unless there is a substantial volume (>45 ml) of infarcted
brain tissue.
   The clinical features are presumed to be related to focal neuronal loss
rather than to neurotransmitter-specific damage.

Clinical features
There is a different clinical history from Alzheimer dementia: usually
there is an account of a sudden deterioration in cognitive performance
or an episode of hemiparesis. Sudden defined strokes or transient
ischaemic attacks (TIAs) followed by a step-wise progression of the
dementia are the hallmark. There is a predominance of focal signs (e.g.
hemiparesis, hemianopia, dysphasia), and pseudobulbar palsy is
common. Bilateral pyramidal signs, 'marche à petits pas', may occur.
Personality, judgement and insight are usually relatively spared.
Emotional incontinence (labile affect, mood swings) occurs frequently.
   Hachinski and his colleagues have included some of the characteristic
features of multi-infarct dementia in a scoring system which can be used
for differentiating multi-infarct dementia from Alzheimer dementia. Table
5.2 shows Hachinski's ischaemic score. Patients with a score of 7 or more
are rated as probable multi-infarct dementia; those with a score of 4 or
below as Alzheimer-type dementia. Exceptions to this demarcation are to
be found in clinical practice, and the number and clinical extent of
strokes, the amount of infarcted tissue seen on CT scan of the brain

38 MANUAL OF GERIATRIC MEDICINE

Table 5.2 The Hachinski ischaemic score

Feature	Score
Abrupt onset	2
Step-wise deterioration	1
Fluctuating course	2
Nocturnal confusion	1
Relative preservation of personality	1
Depression	1
Somatic complaints	1
Emotional incontinence	1
History of hypertension	1
History of strokes	2
Evidence of associated atherosclerosis	1
Focal neurological symptoms	2
Focal neurological signs	2

Interpretation of score:
$\geq$ 7 probable MID
$\leq$ 4 probable Alzheimer dementia
4–7 probable combined MID + Alzheimer dementia

Hachinski V C, Iliff L D, Zilhka E 1975 Cerebral blood flow in dementia. Archives of Neurology 32: 632–637.

and the presence of pseudobulbar palsy should be taken into account. In a study by Rosen et al (1980) of elderly demented patients who came to autopsy, the score has been shown to identify accurately patients with multi-infarct dementia or with mixed pathology.

Prognosis
The risk factors for vascular disease generally include hypertension, cigarette smoking, diabetes, raised blood lipid levels.

Ostfeldt (1980) reported, in a review, that heart disease, hypertension (in particular systolic when diastolic is normal) and diabetes represent risk factors for stroke, but that there was no evidence for an association with cigarette smoking or raised blood lipid levels. However, *not* all individuals who have had a stroke or succession of strokes are demented. The clinical features which increase an individual's risk for multi-infarct dementia have not been clearly identified.

A study by Ladurner et al (1982) addressed this issue, comparing 40 demented stroke patients with 31 stroke patients without dementia. The incidence of hypertension, cardiac disease and diabetes was higher in the demented stroke patients, but only hypertension was significantly higher ($p > 0.001$). There was no difference in viscosity or fibrinogen in the two groups.

Early correction of risk factors, principally hypertension, may prevent progression in some cases and improve prognosis in others in whom the condition is not too advanced.

Subcortical dementia

This term has been applied to the cognitive impairment seen in diseases of cerebral subcortical structures, such as Parkinson's disease, Huntington's chorea and progressive supranuclear palsy. The clinical syndrome consists of acquired intellectual impairment with features of forgetfulness and slowing of mental processes as the primary abnormality; the intellectual deterioration is characterized by difficulty in manipulating acquired knowledge; there are also personality and affective changes, including apathy and depression.

Huntington's chorea

This disorder generally presents between age 30 and 50; there is usually a clear pattern of autosomal dominant inheritance.

Progressive supranuclear palsy

This multi-system disorder is not uncommon in the elderly and may present as parkinsonism. The classic features include
— Eye movement disorder with early involvement of downward gaze (versus involvement of upward gaze in idiopathic parkinsonism), associated with
  ● Nuchal and axial rigidity
  ● Bradykinesia
  ● Gait disorder
  ● A characteristic dysarthria
  ● Progressive dementia
Corticospinal and cerebellar signs may occur; antiparkinsonian drugs are not of any consistent value.

Pick's disease

This pathological curiosity is characterized by asymmetrical lobar atrophy, especially of the frontal lobes and the anterior portion of the temporal lobes. Histologically, there is neuronal loss, gliosis and the presence of argyrophilic inclusion bodies (Pick's bodies), but senile plaques, neurofibrillary tangles and granulovacuolar degeneration are usually lacking.

The clinical symptoms are memory loss, impaired judgement, and confusion, sometimes preceded by lack of energy and blunting of emotions. Progressive decline in memory and cognitive functions is followed by death after a period variously reported as ranging from 2 to 10 years. There are no specific clinical features to differentiate it from Alzheimer dementia, and final diagnosis may have to await post-mortem examination.

Creutzfeldt–Jakob disease

This slow viral encephalopathy results in a rapidly progressive dementia with myoclonus, extrapyramidal signs and multifocal cortical symptoms, leading to death within a few months. There is profound neuronal loss, astrocytosis, and a characteristic spongiform degeneration throughout the brain. It was the first dementing disease shown to be due to a transmissible virus; it usually becomes manifest between the ages of 40 and 60 years, but cases as young as 21 years and as old as 79 years have been described.

Diagnosis of dementia

Most clinicians do not think that brain biopsy is ethically justified for the diagnosis of dementia at present, since there is no specific treatment available.

Essentially the diagnosis of dementia is made on
  1. The history
      a. Subjective complaints about cognitive problems may or may not be present according to the amount of insight retained
      b. The information in the history must always be corroborated by an informant who knows the patient well, especially with regard to evidence of failing intellectual or social capacity, and behavioural evidence
      c. Duration of cognitive impairment, type of onset and type of deterioration are important factors for the differential diagnosis between Alzheimer dementia and acute confusional state, and for the distinction between Alzheimer dementia and multi-infarct dementia
  2. Physical examination and observation of behaviour
  3. Exclusion of other disorders supported by ancillary investigations. Chapter 22 discusses the possible causes of confusion in the elderly and lists ancillary investigations to be applied

CT scan of the brain is sometimes useful in the diagnosis of dementia, but again the pick-up rate of reversible disorders is small. Cerebral atrophy on the scan occurs in intellectually normal old people, but ventricular dilatation is considered to be proportional to the degree of dementia, and appreciable dilatation suggests the presence of normal pressure hydrocephalus. CT scan may support the diagnosis of multi-infarct dementia (i.e. local changes). Its main value is in the detection of potentially treatable lesions such as subdural haematoma, normal pressure hydrocephalus or brain tumour; however, the number of patients in whom treatment significantly improves mental state in the longer term is small (about 2% of all demented patients).

Positron-emission tomographic (PET) scanning has shown that oxygen utilization is reduced in both Alzheimer and multi-infarct dementia, but this is more generalized in Alzheimer dementia, compared with the patchy change in multi-infarct dementia; these features are more pronounced in the grey matter. In Alzheimer dementia the reduced oxygen utilization is due to the reduced oxygen requirements of ailing neurons, whereas in multi-infarct dementia relatively healthy neurons are being starved of oxygen by an impoverished blood supply.

Nuclear magnetic resonance imaging and techniques using evoked potentials may improve diagnosis and are being investigated, with some promising early results.

4. Use of psychometric tests, which are part of the total assessment; certainly, a patient should never be labelled 'demented' on the basis of these tests alone. Aims of psychometric tests are
   a. To differentiate between dementia and depression (see Table 5.4)
   b. To identify diminished cognitive function and to reveal deterioration with time, without which a diagnosis of dementia cannot be made; especially in early stages of dementia impairment of memory and cognitive function may be too subtle to be revealed by psychometric testing; follow-up over time is required; the term 'early dementia' must refer to the earliest stage at which the changes in cognition and behaviour satisfy the criteria for diagnosis of dementia
   c. To make decisions in relation to management

Mental status questionnaires have an evident, though coarse, value in assessing mental competence in the elderly; the 10- or 12-item questionnaires appear to be at least as adequate as the longer versions and are particularly useful as a brief measure that can be easily repeated (see also Ch. 22).

— If a patient obtains a normal score on a mental status questionnaire, but there is strong suspicion of cognitive impairment, more extensive psychometric tests must be done
— Further attention needs to be paid to sensitivity and to the development of tests with a high degree of test–retest reliability
— The problem of measuring change prospectively has not received the attention it deserves

Essentially, the steps towards a diagnosis are the same as for acute confusional state (see Ch. 22). An acute confusional state may be superimposed on dementia and underlying pathology must be sought and treated in order to minimize the risk of further brain damage. The list of conditions associated with acute confusional states in the elderly is shown in Table 22.1. However, there is a very low prevalence of treatable disorders in dementia, and the practical value of applying screening tests routinely to unselected patients is dubious and needs to be evaluated. The role of vitamin B_{12} and folic acid deficiency as a possible cause of dementia is uncertain (post or propter).

Differential diagnosis

— Differential diagnosis of dementia is with acute confusional state (Ch. 22) and depression (Ch. 6)

— Aspects of differential diagnosis between Alzheimer dementia and multi-infarct dementia are shown in Table 5.3

— 'Pseudodementia' is the term that has been applied to the impairment of cognitive function due to depressive illness; psychometric tests reveal impairment of cognitive function which improves with successful treatment of the depression. Other points to distinguish between Alzheimer dementia and depression are shown in Table 5.4

Table 5.3 Differential diagnosis between Alzheimer dementia and multi-infarct dementia

Alzheimer dementia	Multi-infarct dementia
Women more commonly affected	Men more commonly affected
Slow insidious onset	Acute onset with sudden deterioration of cognitive performance or episode of hemiparesis
Gradually progressive deterioration	'Step-wise' deterioration
No focal neurological signs until later stages	Predominance of focal neurological signs
Affect blunted	Affective changes, such as emotional imbalance, depression, anxiety
Personality changes	Personality usually well preserved
Insight lost early	Insight relatively well preserved
Somatic complaints rare	Somatic complaints common
Little evidence of generalized atheromatous disease	Evidence of generalized atheromatous disease often present
Hypertension and convulsions rare	Hypertension and convulsions more common
Hachinski ischaemic score ≤ 4	Hachinski ischaemic score ≥ 7
Senile plaques and neurofibrillary tangles present	Absent
Deficiency of several neurotransmitter systems, especially of the cholinergic neurotransmitter system	No neurotransmitter-specific damage
CT scan shows appreciable ventricular dilatation	CT scan shows local changes, particularly in the temporal regions
PET scan shows generalized reduction in oxygen utilization	PET scan shows patchy reduction in oxygen utilization

Table 5.4 Distinction between depression and Alzheimer dementia

Depression	Alzheimer dementia
History of psychiatric illness of similar kind common	Previous psychiatric history unusual
Rapid onset, often causal link identifiable	Slow insidious onset
Informants are usually aware of the presence of memory and orientation defects	Relatives are frequently unaware of the patient's cognitive defects
Patient complains of cognitive loss; complaints are detailed and often magnified	Patient has little or no complaints of cognitive loss; complaints are usually vague
Patient makes little effort to perform tasks; frequent losses in social and domestic skills	Patient struggles to perform tasks; social skills well preserved until dementia is quite advanced
Patient does not try to keep up	Patient relies on notes, diary and calendar to keep up
Pervasive affective change	Affect shallow
Usually intact speech	Speech disorders frequent
'Don't know' answers and 'can't remember' answers frequent	'Near miss' and wrong answers frequent
Marked variability in performing tasks of similar difficulty	Consistent poor performance on tasks of similar difficulty
Presence of vegetative symptoms characteristic of depression (e.g. insomnia, early morning awakenings, loss of appetite)	Absence of such symptoms
Improvement of results of psychometric tests after treatment with antidepressants	No improvement of results of psychometric tests after treatment with antidepressants
EEG normal	Frequently abnormal

— Benign senile forgetfulness is a relatively stable condition which appears to be associated with memory loss in the absence of other evidence of dementia. The person may recall things on one occasion but not on another; he is aware of his memory loss. The condition can remain stable for many years and institutionalization is not usually required

Treatment

The finding of a specific deficit in the cholinergic system of patients with Alzheimer dementia initially raised hope that a treatment might be found to reverse or halt the progress of the disease. However, therapeutic trials with precursors of acetylcholine have been disappointing. The exploration of pharmacological approaches to correction of this deficit continues.

Other drugs now marketed for use in the treatment of dementias, such as vasodilators, cerebral metabolic enhancers (co-dergocrine, cyclandelate, piracetam) and peptides (vasopressin and some of its analogues such as desmopressin) have proven unsuccessful. Although vasopressin and desmopressin administered intranasally have been found to enhance learning and memory in both demented and healthy persons, the peripheral effects (e.g. water retention, hypertension, tachycardia) proved a serious disadvantage.

At present, drugs are used primarily for symptomatic treatment of, for example, restlessness, agitation, sleep disorders, depression. The minimal effective dose should be used. It is best to be familiar with a small number of well-tried drugs. The continuous supervision of this medication is essential.

Management
Early diagnosis of dementia is likely to improve management of patients and to prevent crisis admissions to hospital (Fig. 5.2). The two major aims of care should be maintenance of the patient's socialization and provision of support for the family or main carer(s). Although reality orientation may be worthwhile, reminiscence group therapy has been found to be most useful in maintaining socialization and establishing group cohesiveness; even patients with severe deficits can respond to familiar social activities and familiar music.

Management of wandering patients includes
— Actions aimed at ensuring safety and security for the patient (such as appropriate lighting, i.e. night lights in bedroom, corridor, toilet)

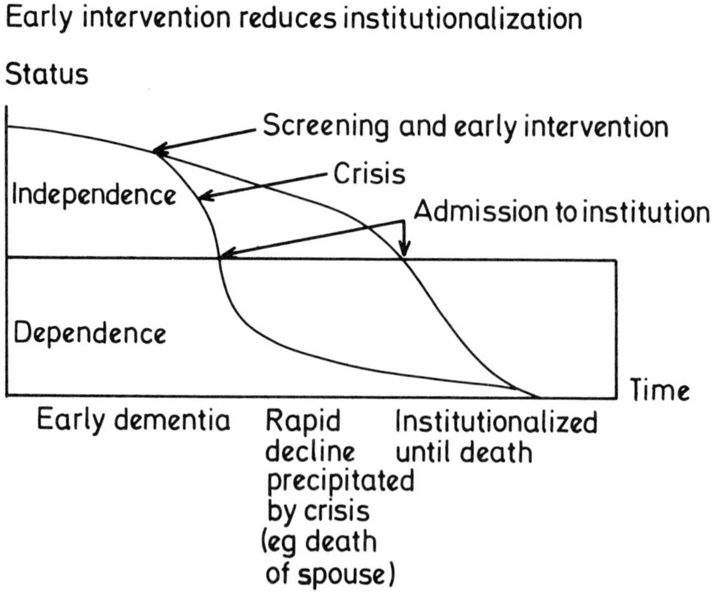

Fig. 5.2 Early intervention reduces institutionalization. Adapted from Bergmann (1982)

— Use of orientation aids: large pictorial signs or symbols are often better than the written word
— Provision of activity, exercise and companionship may prevent wandering occurring

Whenever possible, time spent on explanation and discussion of the management plan with family and/or main carers is invaluable to create understanding, tolerance and support. Relative support groups have been shown to promote insight and good morale. Relief for relatives and/or main carers can be provided by the patient attending at a psychogeriatric day hospital, by relief admissions, and by informing relatives/carers that long-term care will be provided when it can no longer be avoided.

• In some areas Social Services provide an outreach resource which enables home sitters to befriend the elderly confused
• Leaflets and information for relatives and carers are provided by the Alzheimer Disease Society; the most widely used instructional manual, *The 36-Hour Day*, is warmly recommended

BIBLIOGRAPHY

Bergmann K 1982 A community psychiatric approach to the care of the elderly. Are there opportunities for prevention? In: Magnussen G, Nielson J, Buch J (eds) Epidemiology and prevention of mental illness in old age. EGV; Hellerup, Denmark. pp 87–92
Bondareff W 1983 Age and Alzheimer disease. Lancet 1: 1447
Hachinski V C, Iliff L D, Zilhka E 1975 Cerebral blood flow in dementia. Archives of Neurology 32: 632–637
Ladurner G, Iliff L D, Lechner H 1982 Clinical factors associated with dementia in ischaemic stroke. Journal of Neurology, Neurosurgery and Psychiatry 45: 97–101
Mace N L, Rabins P V 1981 The 36-hour day: a family guide to caring for persons with Alzheimer's disease. Johns Hopkins University Press, Baltimore. UK edition 1985 Castleton B (ed). Hodder & Stoughton, Sevenoaks
Ostfeldt A M 1980 A review of stroke epidemiology. Epidemiologic Review 2: 136–152
Report of the Royal College of Physicians on Organic Mental Impairment in the Elderly 1981 Journal of the Royal College of Physicians of London 15: 4–29
Rosen W G, Terry R D, Fuld P A, Katzman R, Peck A 1980 Pathological verification of ischemic score in differentiation of dementias. Annals of Neurology 7: 486–488
Rossor M N, Iversen L L, Johnson A L, Mountjoy C Q, Roth M 1981 The cholinergic defect of the frontal cortex in Alzheimer's disease is age dependent. Lancet 2: 1422
Rossor M N 1982 Neurotransmitters and CNS disease: Dementia. Lancet 2: 1200–1203
Rossor M N, Iversen L L, Reynolds G P, Mountjoy C Q, Roth M 1984 Neurochemical characteristics of early and late onset types of Alzheimer's disease. British Medical Journal 288: 961–964
Tagliavini F, Pilleri G 1983 Neuronal counts in basal nucleus of Meynert in Alzheimer disease and in simple senile dementia. Lancet 1: 469–470
Thompson M K 1985 Myths about the care of the elderly. Lancet 1: 523
Tomlinson B E, Blessed G, Roth M 1970 Observations on the brains of demented old people. Journal of the Neurological Sciences 11: 205–242
Van der Cammen T J M, Simpson J M, Fraser R M, Preker A S, Exton-Smith A N 1987 The Memory Clinic: a new approach to the detection of dementia. British Journal of Psychiatry 150: 359–364

6. DEPRESSION

Definition of a major depressive episode

According to diagnostic criteria DSM-III-R (1987) at least five of the following symptoms should be present during the same 2-week period and represent a change from previous functioning: at least symptom (1) or (2) should be included in order to make the diagnosis

1. Depressed mood most of the day
2. Markedly diminished interest or pleasure in all, or almost all, activities
3. Significant weight loss or weight gain, or decrease or increase in appetite
4. Insomnia or hypersomnia
5. Psychomotor agitation or retardation
6. Fatigue or loss of energy
7. Feelings of worthlessness or excessive or inappropriate guilt (which may be delusional)
8. Diminished ability to think or concentrate, or indecisiveness
9. Recurrent thoughts of death (not just fear of dying), recurrent suicidal ideation without a specific plan, or a suicide attempt or a specific plan for committing suicide.

In addition

— It cannot be established that an organic factor initiated and maintained the disturbance
— The disturbance is not a normal reaction to the death of a loved one (uncomplicated bereavement)
— At no time during the disturbance have there been delusions or hallucinations for as long as 2 weeks in the absence of prominent mood symptoms (i.e. before the mood symptoms developed or after they have remitted)
— Not superimposed on schizophrenia, schizophreniform disorder, delusional disorder or psychotic disorder

Again according to DSM-III-R a mild depressive disorder has few, if any, symptoms in excess of those required to make the diagnosis, and symptoms result in only minor impairment in occupational functioning or in usual social activities or relationships with others.

The term 'minor depressive or dysphoric disorders' has been applied to patients exhibiting three or fewer criteria of major depression. Gillis

& Zabow (1982) found that elderly dysphorics showed marked personal and social isolation, signs of poor coping behaviour and difficult interpersonal relationships. By contrast, the elderly depressives were characterized far more often by previous clear-cut depressions.

For the causation of dysphoria innate or long-standing personality factors seemed to be indicated.

Epidemiology

Depression is the most common form of mental illness in the elderly, its prevalence rising with increasing age. In the world literature, epidemiological studies show 15–20% of subjects over the age of 65 to be suffering from depressive illness, with about 2.5–3.7% of the over 65s suffering from severe or major depression.

A recent study by Copeland et al (1987) found 11.3% of the over-65s living in the Liverpool community to suffer from depressive illness, with 3% suffering from severe depression, while levels for neurotic disorder reached 2.4%.

Suicide attempts are rare in old age; suicidal 'gestures' and ideation need to be taken seriously and should not be dismissed as 'manipulative'.

The vast majority of suicides and parasuicides in old age appear to be associated with a depressive illness rather than a 'rational' decision to end an unbearable situation. Other factors shown to be contributory are social isolation and serious physical illness.

Aetiology

Depressive illness is not based on a single pathology, but has a multifactorial aetiology. In old age, where environmental stresses are so important in bringing about depression, and the adaptability of the personality is diminished, the outlook for depressive illness is less favourable than in younger patients.

— Frequent relapses, incomplete recovery and chronic intractable agitation and gloom are much more common in depression of old age than in younger age groups.
— Genetic factors are less important in late-onset depressions than in depressive illnesses recurring from an earlier age.
— Post (1972) showed that a favourable outcome of depression was associated with
  - Age < 70 years
  - A family history of manic or depressive illness
  - A previous history of severe depression (with full recovery) before the age of 50
  - An extrovert personality and an even temperament
— Bad outcome was associated with
  - Age > 70 years and an aged appearance
  - Any serious, disabling physical illness
  - A history of uninterrupted depression for over 2 years
  - Evidence of brain damage, i.e. neurological signs of dementia

Cole & Hickie (1976) found that greater age, later onset of depression and the presence of minor organic signs were associated with less favourable outcome of the depression; they also found that elderly depressives do not unduly frequently develop dementia.

Cawley et al (1973) found that many elderly depressives have deficits on certain cognitive and neuropsychological tests and that these return to normal less completely in late-onset cases after remission of the depression.

Murphy (1982) found an association between severe life events, major social difficulties, poor physical health and the onset of depression. New was the discovery of the special vulnerability to depression of old people lacking, not so much close and frequent human contacts, but at least one confiding relationship. The lack of such a confidant appeared a reflection of life-long personality traits.

After one year of follow-up only one-third of the elderly depressed patients had a good outcome. Poor outcome was associated with severity of initial depression, those with depressive delusions having a particularly poor outcome. Outcome was also influenced by physical health problems and severe life events in the follow-up year. There was no evidence that an intimate relationship protected against relapse in the face of continuing life stress.

Depression and neurotransmitters

From monoamine research there are strong indications that central monoamine metabolism can be disturbed in depressions and that these disturbances are causal.

In the brain the principal monoamines that function as neurotransmitters are 5-hydroxytryptamine (5-HT, serotonin) and the catecholamines noradrenaline and dopamine. These monoamines have been found to be consistently decreased in the brains of depressed patients. Interest in correlation between monoamines and depression was stimulated by the finding that first-generation antidepressant drugs enhance the availability of 5-HT and noradrenaline at central receptors. The second-generation antidepressants fit this hypothesis too. The third generation (monoamine precursors, selective reuptake inhibitors, postsynaptic agonists) were developed as a result of biological research in depression.

The most widely used antidepressants block the reuptake of noradrenaline and/or 5-HT and, to a lesser extent, of dopamine (except for nomifensine, which inhibits the reuptake of noradrenaline and dopamine equally).

Diagnosis

The history is of paramount importance and should be aimed at eliciting a change from previous functioning and the presence of five or more symptoms of depression as listed in the definition of a major depressive episode. An interview with a relative or another close informant is often useful.

Common symptoms of depression in the elderly may include apathy and withdrawal instead of clear dysphoria, as well as memory impairment, attentional disturbances and significant cognitive deterioration.

Loss of previous interests, activities, appetite and sleep may be difficult to elicit. Though sleep in the elderly may be briefer and more interrupted than in younger persons, elderly depressives, like younger patients, report both early waking and sleep onset difficulties. In contrast to normal elderly, those with depression have been found to exhibit sleep EEGs with considerable shortening in REM latency, reduced sleep efficiency, and an increased number of shifts and arousals throughout the night.

Pitfalls of diagnosis
In the elderly, three factors may lead to underdiagnosis of depression
1. Physical illness may invalidate physical depressive features, such as weight loss and fatigue
2. Elderly patients often minimize feelings of sadness and instead become physically preoccupied
3. Anxiety, obsessionality, hysteria or hypochondriasis of recent onset are often caused by underlying depression, yet such neurotic complaints may obscure the depression. If hypochondriasis is the prominent feature, admission may in the first instance be to a medical or surgical ward (for investigation of constipation, for example)
4. Coexisting social problems may colour the presentation of depression

Pseudodementia
This term has been applied to the impairment of cognitive function due to depressive illness and is a feature frequently encountered in elderly patients with the more severe kinds of affective illness (see also Ch. 5).

Differential diagnosis
Differential diagnosis is with other psychiatric conditions which may show depressive features, and these include organic brain syndromes and paranoid illnesses. Some physical illnesses may present with features initially suggestive of depression, for example hypothyroidism.

Depression rating scales
There is considerable controversy about the use of depression rating scales in the elderly. Good command of language is required; the scales cannot be used when the patient has cognitive impairment. The most frequently used scales at present are the Geriatric Depression Scale (GDS) and the Hamilton Rating Scale (HRS).

Treatment
Drug therapy is not the only line of treatment: psychological treatment, social management and prevention all have important roles. When depression is diagnosed, the severity and symptom pattern are relevant

for management. Most depressed elderly patients are managed in the community by their general practitioner and the associated community health services. Community nurses may be important for providing psychological support and supervising treatment and medication prescribed. Undertreatment of depression in old age is probably common, and a study by Macdonald (1986) showed that general practitioners recognized late-life depression, but such recognition appeared to be unaccompanied by referral to a psychiatrist or treatment with antidepressants.

   — Referral to a psychiatrist may be appropriate in the following circumstances
- Serious diagnostic problems
- Serious suicidal risk
- Severe self-neglect
- Severe agitation, delusions and hallucinations
- Failure to respond to or comply with treatment regimen
- Need to arrange day hospital or in-patient treatment or special services such as community psychiatric nurse or clinical psychology

Antidepressant drugs

Some general rules for prescribing antidepressant medication in the elderly are

   — Choose a sedative drug for agitated/anxious patients
   — Choose a less sedative drug for more retarded patients
   — Night-time dosage may prevent the use of hypnotics
   — As a general rule, antidepressant medication should be started at 25–50% of the normal adult dose, and increased by 25% of the initial dose every 5 days until a therapeutic dosage is obtained and there is stabilization of side effects
   — Watch out for non-compliance: slow onset of action and unpleasant side effects may result in premature cessation of treatment
   — Treatment should be continued for 4–6 weeks at therapeutic doses before the patient is regarded as a non-responder

Tricyclic antidepressants and related drugs

   — These are usually the drugs of first choice (Table 6.1)
   — In the elderly, the newer antidepressants may be preferable because of the lower incidence of anticholinergic side effects; also, they are claimed to be less cardiotoxic in the elderly, but this has not been proven. They may be tried in patients with contraindications to tricyclic antidepressants, but only with extreme caution and under close supervision; careful cardiac monitoring is required for patients who have cardiac arrhythmias
   — The efficacy of tricyclic antidepressants is well established; however, a proportion of patients (estimated at one-third) do not respond; others have only a partial response

Table 6.1 Examples of antidepressant drugs

Tricyclic antidepressants	
Sedating	Amitriptyline
	Dothiepin
Less sedating	Imipramine
	Nortriptyline
Stimulating	Protriptyline
Newer antidepressants	
Sedating	Trazodone
	Mianserin
Less sedating	Maprotiline
	Lofepramine
	Fluvoxamine

Monoamine oxidase inhibitors Phenelzine

— Usually, insomnia and anxiety symptoms improve first; other symptoms may not show consistent improvement for 10–14 days
— Amitriptyline and imipramine are two established tricyclic antidepressants against which newer drugs have been compared
— Side effects of tricyclic antidepressants and allied drugs are
  • Anticholinergic: dry mouth, constipation, micturition difficulty, blurred vision (visual accommodation problems)
  • Cardiovascular: cardiac arrhythmias, cardiac failure, postural hypotension
  • Gastrointestinal: nausea
  • Neurological: drowsiness, epilepsy, tremor
  • Psychiatric: confusional state
  • Haematological: neutropenia, agranulocytosis
— Absolute contraindications are prostatism and glaucoma. Cardiac disease, especially cardiac arrhythmia, is a relative contraindication

Lithium

— Lithium is of some value in preventing or reducing the frequency of recurrences of manic depression
— A psychiatric opinion should be sought before starting an elderly patient on lithium
— Dosage must be lowered in the elderly because of a reduced renal clearance and decreased volume of distribution; serum levels are inversely related to both glomerular filtration rate (GFR) and volume distribution
— The narrow therapeutic range makes regular plasma monitoring necessary; this should be accompanied by careful clinical evaluations
— Great caution is necessary in patients with heart disease
— Serious CNS symptoms may occur in lithium intoxication

and include: memory impairment, confusion, agitation, drowsiness, dysarthria, ataxia
— Electrolyte imbalance, especially of sodium, may result in lithium toxicity
— Side effects include
  • Anorexia,* vomiting,* diarrhoea*
  • Tremor*
  • Polyuria with polydipsia
  • Hypothyroidism
*These are warning signs of incipient toxicity
— Contraindications are renal failure and recent myocardial infarction

Monoamine oxidase inhibitors
These drugs are not often used in old people because of the high frequency of adverse drug reactions, and the risk of severe hypertensive crises occurring when patients take substances such as ephedrine, amphetamines, tyramine.

A psychiatric opinion should be sought before starting an elderly person on an MAOI. They are potentially indicated in patients with life-long histories of characterological depression accompanied by high levels of anxiety.

ECT
If depression does not respond to medical treatment or the number and severity of side effects are intolerable, electroconvulsive therapy (ECT) should be considered; it is considered to be particularly beneficial in severe depession when biological features are prominent or depressive psychosis is evident. It is usually given twice a week up to a total of between four and eight sessions. A degree of memory loss for recent events may follow ECT, but this usually clears within 1–3 months.

With improvement in drug treatments, it is likely that patients who will be receiving ECT will include a higher proportion with very refractory illness, and future outcome evaluations must take this into account.

Prevention
— Prevention of (recurrent) depression may be achieved in some patients by maintaining social adjustment and activities, although the personality of the subject may be a limiting factor
— Effective treatment of physical illness may be useful in avoiding another precipitating factor. Also, reassurance about the patient's physical condition may help to alleviate the depression
— Finally, it is important to support any confiding relationships as far as possible

BIBLIOGRAPHY

American Psychiatric Association 1987 Diagnostic and statistical manual of mental disorders, 3rd edn (revised). APA, Washington, DC

Blazer D, Williams C D 1980 Epidemiology of dysphoria and depression in an elderly population. American Journal of Psychiatry 137: 439–444

Cawley R H, Post F, Whitehead A 1973 Barbiturate tolerance and psychological functioning in elderly depressed patients. Psychological Medicine 1: 39–52

Cole M, Hickie R N 1976 Frequency and significance of minor organic signs in elderly depressives. Canadian Psychiatric Association Journal 21: 7–12

Copeland J R M, Dewey M E, Wood N, Searle R, Davidson I A, McWilliam C 1987 Range of mental illness among the elderly in the community: Prevalence in Liverpool using the GMS–AGECAT package. British Journal of Psychiatry 150: 815–823

Fraser R M, Glass I B 1980 Unilateral and bilateral ECT in elderly patients. Acta Psychiatrica Scandinavica 62: 13–31

Gillis L S, Zabow A 1982 Dysphoria in the elderly. South African Medical Journal 62: 410–413

Hamilton M 1967 Development of a rating scale for primary depressive illness. British Journal of Social and Clinical Psychology 6: 278–296

Kupfer D J, Spiker D G, Coble P A et al 1978 Electroencephalographic sleep recordings and depression in the elderly. Journal of the American Geriatrics Society 26: 53–57

Macdonald A J D 1986 Do general practitioners 'miss' depression in elderly patients? British Medical Journal 292: 1365–1367

Murphy E 1982 Social origins of depression in old age. British Journal of Psychiatry 141: 135–142

Murphy E 1983 The prognosis of depression in old age. British Journal of Psychiatry 142: 111–119

Post F 1972 The management and nature of depressive illnesses in late life: A follow-through study. British Journal of Psychiatry 121: 393–404

van Praag H M 1982 Neurotransmitters and CNS disease: Depression. Lancet 2: 1259–1264

Yesavage J A, Brink T L, Rose T L, Lum O, Huang V, Adey M, Leirer O 1983 Development and validation of a geriatric depression screening scale: A preliminary report. Journal of Psychiatric Research 17: 37–49

7. SLEEP DISORDERS

Normal sleep

There are two physiological distinct states
- Rapid eye movement sleep (REM) or dreaming
- Deep sleep, slow wave sleep (NREM); this is divided into stages 1–4.

In REM sleep the brain is very active and EEG recordings are similar to those in the waking state. There is subsidence in muscle activity, with the exception of eye movements, and spinal reflexes are lost. In NREM sleep bodily movements are relatively infrequent, although muscle electrical activity and reflex excitability are well maintained.
- When normal adults fall asleep they usually pass directly into NREM sleep. After this, there is regular 90–100-minute alternation between NREM and REM sleep — the basic sleep cycle.

Physiological changes with age

Some of the changes in the overall sleep pattern with age are
- Total nocturnal sleep time diminishes
- Wake periods become more frequent and prolonged
- The number of shifts between sleep periods, particularly to stage 1, is increased
- The total amount of stage 1 sleep increases steadily throughout life
- The percentage of sleep in stage 2 follows a U-shaped curve during life and the levels in old age resemble those in early adult life
- Stage 3 sleep remains relatively unchanged in old age
- Stage 4 sleep shows a relative and absolute reduction from the age of 20 years onwards and by the age of 60 25% of the population have no stage 4 sleep

All these changes correlate with the typical components in old age of less nocturnal sleep, less refreshing sleep and more frequent awakenings. Associated with the reduction in nocturnal sleep many older people have daytime sleepiness with naps lasting 1 hour or more.

— The relative amount of REM sleep remains almost constant
throughout life, with a small decline in extreme old age

Pathological conditions affecting sleep

The elderly are prone to suffer from several physical and psychiatric
disorders which lead to sleep disturbances, and some of these are shown
in Table 7.1.

Table 7.1 Pathological conditions affecting sleep

Sleep apnoea
Nocturnal leg movements
Restless legs syndrome
Night cramp
Pain in arthritis and musculoskeletal disorders
Bodily discomfort due to distended bladder and rectum, and oesophageal reflux
Nocturia
Psychophysiological insomnia
Depression
Organic mental deterioration
Drug-related insomnia

Sleep apnoea

— Sleep apnoea consists of a nocturnal sleep disturbance
characterized by a cessation of air-flow with subsequent
arousal. It probably affects 40% of old people even though
they may be unaware of the cause or the recurrence of
sleep disturbance
— There are two forms, obstructive and central, although a
mixed type with predominance of obstruction also occurs. In
obstructive apnoea the airway is occluded by soft tissue of
the oropharynx, resulting in reduced air exchange
(hypoapnoea) followed by respiratory effort, snoring and
bodily movements. In central apnoea the stimulus to
respiration is lost and there is no respiratory effort
— As a consequence of the sleep disturbances drowsiness in
the daytime almost invariably occurs. This may be small,
amounting to a nap in quiet sedentary moments, or very
debilitating with severe daytime somnolence
— Any older person who suffers from daytime somnolence and
snoring should be suspected as having sleep apnoea. The
diagnosis can be made by a night-time observer or by the
use of a cassette recorder switched on at bedtime. Sleep
apnoea must be distinguished from Cheyne–Stokes
respiration

Nocturnal leg movements

— Nocturnal leg movements are a common cause of difficulty
in maintaining sleep. These movements are varied but often

consist of periodic extension of the big toe, flexion of the foot at the ankle and flexion of the knee and hip. The movements may be unilateral or bilateral, and confined to the early part of the night or recurring throughout the night

— The relationship between these movements and frequent awakening and arousal is well documented. The cause of the condition is unknown and there is no proven effective treatment

Restless leg syndrome (see p. 181)

Night cramp (see p. 181)

Pain

Pain of almost any description can disturb sleep. Most commonly in the elderly it is due to osteoarthritis; associated with pain in the knees may be sudden jerky movements of the joints. In cervical spondylosis there may be pain as well as distressing paraesthesiae in the upper limbs. If possible, pain should be controlled by analgesics before hypnotics are given.

— Bodily discomfort from distended viscera, such as distension of the bladder, loading of the rectum and oesophageal reflux, are important causes of restlessness at night and insomnia.

Nocturia

Nocturia is one of the commonest physical complaints in the elderly giving rise to insomnia. In severe cases the patient may get up four or more times at night to pass urine. Water excretion is delayed in old age and fluid taken before retiring may not be excreted until 3–4 hours later.

Depression

Characteristically, the type of insomnia in depression is 'early morning wakening' — the patient wakes up at 3 or 4 a.m. and has difficulty in getting back to sleep. The depth and the total amount of sleep are reduced.

Alzheimer's disease

There is often a polyphasic sleep cycle with frequent naps distributed throughout the day. Nocturnal sleep is brief and frequently fragmented by numerous awakenings.

Drug-induced sleep disorders

Chronic use of sedative hypnotics, alcohol and caffeine are responsible for insomnia in many old people. The connection between insomnia and the drinking of coffee in the evening is often not recognized.

Parkinsonian patients may have sleep disturbances related to the illness and more commonly to the drugs used to treat them. Bromocriptine and L-dopa with dopa decarboxylase inhibitors may induce nightmares along with mild toxic reactions presenting as confusion and wandering.

Hypnotics

— One of the commonest causes of insomnia is the long-term use of hypnotics which disrupt nocturnal sleep. Habituation leads some patients to increase the dose in an attempt to maintain or restore the therapeutic effect. Physical and psychological dependence follows the development of tolerance. Sleep continuity is disrupted in the second part of the night owing to loss of effectiveness.

— A study of the subjective qualities of sleep in elderly patients attending a geriatric day hospital has shown that the frequency of night-time awakenings was greatest and the quality of sleep was judged to be poorer in those who took hypnotics compared with those who did not (Gerard et al 1978).

— In one study of a random sample of old people living at home in a London borough (Exton-Smith 1977) 28% took hypnotics regularly (35% of females and 24% of males) and 26% took hypnotics nightly.

— The use of nocturnal sedation has significant adverse effects by increasing the arousal threshold, impairing balance and the production of anterograde insomnia for night-time events. In consequence there may be decreased ability to respond to emergency situations, with increased nocturnal falls and hip fractures. The widespread prescription of benzodiazepines is creating a serious problem of drug dependence.

Management

Diagnosis

In all cases of insomnia the patient should keep a sleep diary and complete a questionnaire. Although many old people live and sleep alone it is desirable whenever possible to obtain information on the patient's sleep pattern from a partner, because subjective evaluation of sleep is very unreliable. A full history should be obtained and particular attention should be paid to prescribed and over-the-counter drugs.

General measures

The patient should try to adhere to the following rules

1. Keep a set wake-up time on weekdays and at weekends
2. Avoid daytime naps or restrict to half an hour in the afternoon at the most
3. Avoid the regular use of caffeine and alcohol
4. Restrict fluid intake in the evening for at least 4–5 hours before retiring when nocturia is a problem
5. Increased exercise and social activities should be encouraged
6. If the patient is not sleepy when retiring and cannot sleep, he should get up rather than toss and turn about in bed
7. Muscle relaxation techniques under the initial instruction of a physiotherapist can often help to relieve tension which is contributing to insomnia

Hypnotics

Many patients expect the prescription of a 'sleeping pill' for the treatment of their insomnia. It should be explained to them that sleep patterns change in old age; the amount of sleep is reduced and the former patterns of youth cannot be re-established. Hypnotics should only be used on a short-term basis. Owing to altered pharmokinetics the half-life of benzodiazepines is increased in elderly subjects. Long-acting agents such as nitrazepam accumulate after use for 2–3 days and toxicity becomes evident with chronic use. Short-acting benzodiazepines are to be preferred and are less likely to produce hangover. But it has been found that the plasma concentration of 'short-acting' temazepam increases by 50% after 7 days of use.

BIBLIOGRAPHY

Gerard P, Collins K J, Dore C, Exton-Smith A N 1978 Subjective characteristics of sleep in the elderly. Age and Ageing 7 (suppl): 55–59

Morgan K 1987 Sleep and ageing: A research based guide to sleep in later life. Croom-Helm, London

Pascualy R 1985 Sleep disorders. In: Exton-Smith A N, Weksler M (eds) Practical geriatric medicine. Churchill Livingstone, Edinburgh

8. HYPERTENSION

Definition

The WHO definition of hypertension: >160/>95 mmHg appears applicable to the age group of 65–80 years old.

Although about 5% of both men and women aged 65 or over have a systolic blood pressure exceeding 200 mmHg and a diastolic pressure of 100 mmHg or more, the elderly hypertensive is commonly defined as aged 65 or over, with a systolic blood pressure of ≥160 mmHg, a diastolic pressure of ≥95 mmHg, or both.

Introduction

The risk of cardiovascular disease increases with blood pressure at all ages and in both sexes. The risk of stroke and heart failure is especially high in older hypertensive patients. Treating raised blood pressure in the elderly poses problems: they are at especial risk from unwanted effects of drugs and from interactions with drugs taken for other diseases; and, as systolic blood pressure rises with age, partly because the arterial walls lose elasticity, the definition of hypertension in older patients is less certain. The clinical problem is to determine at what level of blood pressure and in which particular patients the benefits from treatment outweigh the disadvantages.

Blood pressure and ageing

Blood pressure increases with age in industrialized societies, so that more than a third of those between the ages of 65 and 74 have pressures of ≥160 mmHg systolic and/or 95 mmHg diastolic. This progressive rise in pressure is actually more accurately described as a persistent rise in systolic pressure.

Diastolic values for the population as a whole tend to peak at about age 45–50 and then plateau; the overall diastolic increase is accounted for by the roughly one-third of the population in which pressures rise. Sever et al (1980) found that in many non-Western societies the tendency of blood pressure to rise with age does not occur and blood pressure tends to be low and remain so throughout life, especially in those organized as hunting and gathering units; the reason is unknown; a genetic cause is unlikely since it has been established that, when residents of these societies migrate to metropolitan centres, their blood pressure tends to rise. Environmental factors, dietary and psychosocial, have been implicated as causes of the inexorable rise of pressure seen in Western societies. However, the exact cause of the phenomenon has not been defined.

Physiological changes occurring with ageing

The widespread utilization of non-invasive techniques for assessing left ventricular performance has facilitated the study of cardiac structure and function in elderly individuals without latent cardiovascular disease.

Senescent changes in human cardiovascular structure and function are shown in Table 8.1; effects of ageing on exercise physiology are shown in Table 8.2 (Walsh 1987).

Due to the reduction in aortic distensibility (Table 8.1, Fig. 8.1), the introduction of a relatively small volume of fluid into the aorta of an elderly individual may significantly increase systolic blood pressure, whereas a minimal reduction in fluid volume in the aorta of an elderly individual may cause a dramatic decrease in blood pressure. Other age-related changes include a reduction in baroreceptor sensitivity, a reduction in plasma renin activity and an increase in plasma norepinephrine levels.

Table 8.1 Senescent changes in human cardiovascular structure and function

Cardiac
  Modest concentric left ventricular hypertrophy and increased left atrial diameter
  Normal systolic function at rest (e.g. ejection fraction)
  Abnormal diastolic filling

Vascular
  Increased aortic diameter and wall thickness
  Decreased aortic elasticity
  Decreased beta-adrenergically mediated systemic arteriolar vasodilation
  Increased aortic impedance during exercise

From Walsh (1987).

Table 8.2 Effects of ageing on exercise physiology

Decreased maximal oxygen consumption
Narrowed overall arteriovenous oxygen difference
Normal cardiac output at peak exercise
Decreased dependence on heart rate and increased reliance upon the Frank–Starling mechanism to augment cardiac output during exercise

From Walsh (1987).

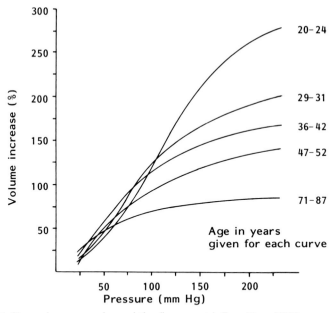

Fig. 8.1 Changes in pressure-volume relation (human aorta). From Moser (1988)

ESSENTIAL HYPERTENSION

Characteristics

Messerli et al (1983) demonstrated that essential hypertension in the elderly constitutes a distinct entity with specific cardiac, haemodynamic, volume and endocrine findings.

Thirty patients with established essential hypertension aged over 65 years were matched for mean arterial pressure, race, sex, height and weight with 30 patients with established essential hypertension younger than 42 years. Cardiac output, heart rate, stroke volume, intravascular volume, renal blood flow and plasma renin activity were significantly lower in the older age group, whereas total peripheral (and renal vascular) resistance, left ventricular posterior wall and septal thicknesses and left ventricular mass were higher. Intravascular volume correlated inversely with total peripheral resistance in both groups and in all patients.

Pathophysiological findings of essential hypertension in the elderly were characterized by a hypertrophied heart of the concentric type with a low cardiac output resulting from a smaller stroke volume and a slower heart rate; renal blood flow was disproportionately reduced and total peripheral and renal vascular resistance elevated.

It was concluded that 'essential hypertension is a pathophysiological process that accelerates the physiological, haemodynamic, fluid volume, and endocrine processes of ageing and thus reflects a faster-running biological clock'.

The risks of hypertension

Essential hypertension is a risk factor for stroke, cardiovascular disease, peripheral arterial disease, renal failure, hypertensive retinopathy and occlusion of the retinal vein.

Ostfeld et al (1971) reported that in the over-65s the 43% with pressures of $\geqslant 160/\geqslant 95$ mmHg had twice the incidence of stroke of those with lower pressures; there was also an increased incidence in congestive cardiac failure and coronary heart disease in this group.

Wilkie & Eisdorfer (1971) reported that cognitive function showed a substantially greater decline over a 10-year period after the age of 60 among elderly hypertensives with evidence of end-organ disease and without treatment, than among normotensive elderly people.

Kannel (1976) reported that elevated blood pressure is the most significant controllable risk factor for cardiovascular disease among the elderly.

There are no hard data defining the prevalence or incidence of renovascular stenosis in the elderly. In older hypertensive patients widespread arteriosclerosis is common, and partial obstruction of a renal artery may be far more frequent than is currently believed.

Retinal changes in elderly hypertensive patients usually combine mild abnormalities of both atherosclerotic and hypertensive origin. Severe hypertensive retinopathy is rare, and suggests a renal or renovascular origin.

ISOLATED SYSTOLIC HYPERTENSION

In patients over 70, isolated systolic hypertension is more prevalent than diastolic hypertension. Colandrea et al (1970) defined isolated systolic hypertension in subjects aged 65 years or over as $>160/<90$ mmHg, while Dyer et al (1977) used $>160/<95$ mmHg. The general opinion at present is that isolated systolic hypertension is diagnosed when the diastolic pressure is less than 90 mmHg and the systolic pressure exceeds 160 mmHg (Gifford 1982).

Isolated systolic hypertension is found in approximately 25–30% of men and women aged over 75.

It is currently unknown whether treatment of isolated systolic hypertension in the elderly is associated with a reduction in risk; the condition is recognized to be associated with a two- to threefold increase in mortality, especially from cardiovascular disease and stroke. Several studies have shown that systolic blood pressure can be safely lowered in the elderly. Further studies are addressing the issue of the value of treatment of isolated systolic hypertension in reducing risk.

Assessment of the elderly hypertensive

History
Previous medical history is especially important with regard to the presence of other risk factors, particularly diabetes mellitus and previous events that may represent hypertensive complications.

Onset of essential hypertension and of malignant hypertension are uncommon in elderly patients. Documentation of normal blood pressures in the recent past or evidence of a malignant form of hypertension will require a more detailed investigation. Otherwise, the diagnosis is likely to be essential hypertension, and a limited number of investigations will suffice.

Symptoms suggesting target organ involvement should be specifically sought.

A detailed drug history is mandatory.

Blood pressure reading
— Blood pressure reading of >160/95 mmHg: systolic plus diastolic hypertension
— Blood pressure reading of >160/<90 mmHg: isolated systolic hypertension (Gifford 1982)

An auscultatory gap is a common finding in elderly hypertensives and may lead to an underestimation of systolic pressure. This can be avoided by inflating the blood pressure cuff until the radial pulse is no longer palpable. Perhaps, because of the loss of elasticity of the arterial tree, there is often no point of disappearance of the Korotkov sounds. Therefore, the point of muffling (phase IV) is often the best approximation of diastolic pressure in the elderly patient.

Variability in blood pressure increases with age; most clinicians rely on two or three blood pressure determinations several weeks apart in order to confirm the diagnosis; blood pressure should be taken on both right and left arm at the level of the heart; the highest value should be used to determine management; blood pressure, before and during treatment, should always be monitored after several minutes of standing, because symptoms of orthostatic hypotension may occur associated with a reduction in systolic blood pressure of as much as 30–40 mmHg after 1 minute of standing (see also Ch. 10).

Damage to target organs
Complications of hypertension occur in the target organs, i. e. the brain, eyes, heart, kidneys, aorta and arterial system.
— Brain: an increased risk of stroke, especially of atherothrombotic stroke, and possibly a decline in cognitive function

— Eyes: development of hypertensive retinopathy; hypertension is also a predisposing factor for retinal vein occlusion
— Heart: left ventricular hypertrophy, left ventricular failure, congestive cardiac failure, coronary artery disease, myocardial infarction, aortic valve sclerosis
  • There is also a higher incidence of left bundle branch block (LBBB) in hypertensive people than in normotensive people
— Kidneys: nephrosclerosis, renal impairment
  • Renal impairment can be arbitrarily divided into three grades (Table 8.3)

Table 8.3

	GFR (ml/min)	Approximate serum creatinine (μ mol/l)
Mild	20–50	150–300
Moderate	10–20	300–700
Severe	<10	>700

— Aorta and arterial system: generalized atherosclerosis, unfolding of the thoracic aorta, aortic calcification, atherosclerotic and/or thrombotic narrowing or occlusion of the abdominal aorta, atherosclerotic aneurysm of the abdominal aorta, peripheral arterial insufficiency

The physical examination should include an assessment of target organ involvement.

This includes a neurological evaluation and fundoscopy.

A laterally displaced or sustained apical impulse suggests cardiac involvement, as does a third heart sound. Increased intensity of the aortic component of the second heart sound implies that at least moderate hypertension has been present for several years. In the absence of left bundle branch block, paradoxical splitting of the second heart sound is rare. Systolic ejection murmurs are common. Early diastolic decrescendo murmurs can occur with hypertension alone and do not necessarily imply independent valvular heart disease. Mitral regurgitation murmurs are commonly due to left ventricular dilatation, but may represent organic mitral valve disease.

The patient may present with left ventricular failure, but if this is mild it may be overlooked by the patient, so that at the time of presentation symptoms and signs of right ventricular failure may predominate.

Bruits should be sought in the abdomen and flanks as well as in the peripheral arteries; the bruit of renal artery stenosis may be heard over the back. Transmitted pulsations in the upper abdomen are indicative of an aneurysm of the abdominal aorta.

Investigations

Essential investigations
- Body weight
- Urinanalysis
- Urea and electrolytes
- Serum creatinine level: a normal serum creatinine level in an elderly person does not mean that renal function is normal: in the elderly muscle mass is low — so serum creatinine level should be quite low; in addition, serum creatinine level does not represent glomerular filtration rate (GFR, creatinine clearance)
- Creatinine clearance: if necessary use the Siersbaek–Nielsen nomogram for rapid bedside evaluation of creatinine clearance. This nomogram relies on 'steady-state' renal function and may only be used where serum creatinine level is less than 400 μmol/l (see also Ch. 30)
- Serum glucose: diabetes mellitus is associated with a higher incidence of hypertension
- Full blood count: low haemoglobin and low red blood count associated with abnormal renal function indicate anaemia secondary to renal impairment
- Total cholesterol and high density lipoprotein are usually normal in elderly hypertensives, but levels may be adversely affected by diuretics or beta-adrenergic blocking agents and thus pretreatment levels should be established
- ECG
- Chest X-ray

Optional investigations
- Echocardiography: can be used to document left ventricular wall thickness and valvular abnormalities
- CT scan of the abdominal aorta may visualize an aneurysm and involvement of the renal arteries

Aspects of treatment

It is generally agreed that patients with evidence of target organ involvement should be treated, even though it may be too late to derive maximum benefit from therapy. Furthermore, evidence from various studies suggests that there is a strong case for treating all elderly hypertensive patients, up to the age of 80 years
- Studies by Rajala et al (1983) suggest that in the over-80s there seems to be an inverse relation between systolic and diastolic blood pressure and 2-year mortality
- The value of treatment of isolated systolic hypertension in reducing risk is the subject of further studies
- The results of the European Working Party on High Blood

Pressure in the Elderly Trial (1985) demonstrated that
elderly patients tolerate antihypertensive medication without
too much difficulty if it is administered in relatively small
doses and management is kept simple; in addition, the
number of cardiac deaths was significantly lower for those
receiving treatment and this included a substantial reduction
in deaths from myocardial infarction; the reduction in
cerebrovascular mortality was appreciable, but statistically
non-significant; however, there was a fall in the rate of
non-fatal cerebrovascular accidents by 52% and this
reduction was statistically significant
— Weight reduction and dietary salt restriction have been
shown to be independently effective in reducing blood
pressure, but the only type of intervention shown to be
associated with a reduction in cardiovascular morbidity is
drug therapy
— The elderly hypertensive patient tends to be more sensitive
to any intervention because of impaired homeostatic
mechanisms
— Treatment should be carefully selected for each individual
patient. Patient compliance is a recognized problem in
antihypertensive therapy, since many hypertensive patients
are asymptomatic; therefore, side effects of treatment
should be minimal and should not reduce the patient's
independence. The choice of the most appropriate drug
depends on the different ancillary properties with regard to
the cardiovascular system and should be based on the
presence of associated damage (i. e. left ventricular failure,
congestive cardiac failure). The presence of other illnesses
(e.g. depression) should also be taken into account
— Lower blood pressure gradually in order to maintain
cerebral blood flow
— Diastolic blood pressure should not reach levels lower than
90 mmHg. Aim for a systolic blood pressure level between
140 and 160 mmHg; if the systolic pressure remains higher
one must accept the systolic pressure that is associated with
the optimal diastolic pressure

Treatment

General

— Weight reduction
— Reduction of salt intake (low-salt diet, not salt-free)
— Stop smoking
— Stop alcohol intake
— Stop drugs which are known to cause hypertension (if at all
possible): oestrogen, progesterone, corticosteroids, liquorice,

amphetamines, sympathomimetics, monoamine oxidase inhibitors

Specific

Medication aimed at decreasing heart work and oxygen demand includes
1. Diuretics (reduce volume overload and blood pressure)
2. Vasodilators, converting enzyme inhibitors or alpha-blockers (reduce afterload)
3. Venodilators (reduce preload)

The above three measures all aim to decrease heart work and oxygen demand.

4. Inotropic agents such as digoxin may be administered to increase cardiac efficiency in patients with associated left ventricular failure or congestive cardiac failure
5. Antiarrhythmic agents may be administered to regulate heart rate
6. Beta-adrenergic inhibitors may be administered to decrease oxygen need
7. Calcium channel blockers may be given to reduce afterload (hypertension) as well as to induce coronary artery vasodilatation

All of these agents (1–7 inclusive) help to relieve the symptoms and signs of the oxygen 'supply and demand imbalance'.

— Pathological processes in the peripheral circulation are usually managed by medications that dilate blood vessels or decrease the oxygen demand of peripheral tissue

Choice of drug

The drugs invariably used first in all clinical trials have been the diuretics — the thiazides and the loop diuretics.

Thiazides

Thiazides act by increasing sodium excretion and reducing plasma volume, contributing to a reduction in cardiac output. They tend to reduce peripheral vascular resistance through total body sodium depletion. They are usually well tolerated and effective in small doses, which are unlikely to aggravate any pre-existing tendency to orthostatic hypotension or to further impair the reflexes that maintain cardiovascular homeostasis. Once-daily dosage will improve compliance. The results of the European Working Party on High Blood Pressure in the Elderly Trial showed a proven beneficial potential for improving the cardiovascular prognosis in the elderly hypertensive, especially when normal serum potassium levels were ensured.

Disadvantages

— Danger of inducing hypokalaemia, hyponatraemia, hypochloraemic alkalosis

Note:

- Intoxication with cardiac glycosides (digoxin) can be induced by hypokalaemia, i.e. serum potassium level <3.5 mmol/l
- When serum potassium is very low, i.e. 1–2 mmol/l, and there is accompanying hypochloraemic alkalosis, hypokalaemic myopathy may develop: this is usually a mainly proximal myopathy: the main symptom is (generalized) muscle weakness; on examination there are depressed deep tendon reflexes

— Danger of inducing hypercalcaemia: thiazide diuretics are potent inhibitors of calcium excretion in the distal tubuli
— Danger of hyperuricaemia: gout may be aggravated

Note:

- Hyperuricaemia alone (without clinical manifestations of gout) does not warrant treatment with allopurinol

— Decreased glucose tolerance: diabetes mellitus can be precipitated or aggravated
— Danger of dehydration (thirst regulation is often impaired in the elderly)
— Orthostatic hypotension and urinary incontinence may be induced or aggravated
— Thiazide diuretics can worsen an already impaired renal function and are ineffective when GFR is below 20 ml/min; they are contraindicated in renal failure; they can cause interstitial nephritis
— In hepatic failure hypokalaemia caused by thiazide diuretics can precipitate encephalopathy
— Acetazolamide, carbenoloxone, corticosteroids and corticotrophin in combination with thiazides increase the risk of hypokalaemia
— Necrotizing vasculitis may occur
— Less common side effects are: skin rashes, photosensitivity, vertigo, nausea, diarrhoea, thrombocytopenia, neutropenia.

Loop diuretics

The loop diuretics, frusemide and ethacrynic acid, are less effective as chronic antihypertensive agents than thiazides and should not be used as antihypertensive agents except in patients with congestive cardiac failure (CCF) or renal failure; because of their rapid action they carry a greater risk of inducing orthostatic hypotension and urinary incontinence; also, there is a greater risk of developing hypokalaemia than with thiazides.

If the therapeutic response to diuretic medication is inadequate, a second drug such as a beta-adrenergic blocking agent, methyldopa, angiotensin converting enzyme inhibitor, vasodilator or calcium channel blocker may be added. Evidence of benefit of these drugs in the treatment of elderly hypertensive patients is awaited and further studies are addressing this issue. The choice of drug should be determined specifically for each individual patient.

Beta-adrenergic blocking agents
Beta-blockers antagonize the actions of catecholamines by competitive inhibition. They act by reducing cardiac output and by inhibiting reflex autonomic activity and renin release from the kidneys. They are effective in angina pectoris and have been shown to be cardioprotective after myocardial infarction. They delay atrioventricular conduction and may therefore be of use in patients with certain heart rhythm disorders (see Ch. 9). They have a negative inotropic effect on the heart muscle and may precipitate congestive cardiac failure. They lessen renal blood flow because they depress cardiac output. Ultimate excretion is usually by the kidneys, so in renal failure the dose may have to be lowered. Fat-soluble beta-blockers permeate the blood–brain barrier and may cause CNS side effects such as vivid dreams, nightmares and depression; both fat- and water-soluble beta-blockers have been found to impair memory function in the elderly. Fat-soluble beta-blockers also have a high hepatic clearance and should be avoided in patients with liver disease.

— Contraindications to the use of beta-blockers include left ventricular and congestive cardiac failure, severe bradycardia, heart block (beyond first degree), 'sick sinus' syndrome, asthma and chronic obstructive pulmonary disease, severe or worsening claudication and gangrene
— Complications of the use of beta-blockers include bradycardia, possible reduction of high-density lipoproteins, peripheral vasospasm and exacerbation of Raynaud's phenomenon
— Sudden withdrawal of a beta-blocker in patients with angina pectoris is dangerous; they should be avoided in non-compliant patients who have angina pectoris.
— Beta-blockers can block the adrenergic symptoms of hypoglycaemia and can delay recovery from hypoglycaemia induced by insulin or oral hypoglycaemic drugs. The clinical importance of these effects is probably small in most diabetics, but beta-blockers are best avoided in unstable diabetics prone to episodes of hypoglycaemia.

Methyldopa
This is an effective antihypertensive drug and is well tolerated by most elderly hypertensives. However, it has potential CNS depressant effects and therefore should be initiated cautiously. The major side effects are sedation, depression and orthostatic hypotension.

A positive direct Coombs' test can occur in up to 20% of patients; this appears to be dose-related and only infrequently associated with a haemolytic anaemia.

Angiotensin converting enzyme inhibitors
(ACE inhibitors: captopril, enalapril). These lower blood pressure

primarily through suppression of the renin–angiotensin–aldosterone system; they are potent vasodilators with favourable haemodynamic effects. They are particularly useful if there is concurrent congestive cardiac failure or a high renin state. They are potassium-saving owing to suppression of aldosterone production, and therefore should not be combined with potassium-saving diuretics or potassium supplements.

ACE inhibitors may be very effective in patients with bilateral renal artery stenoses or renal artery stenosis in a solitary kidney; however, close monitoring of renal function is required and these patients ought to be admitted to hospital for initiation of therapy.

— Contraindications include severe renal impairment with a creatinine clearance below 20 ml/min, serious collagen vascular disease, especially systemic lupus erythematosus (SLE), and use of concomitant medication known to cause neutropenia, e.g. immunosuppressives, cytotoxic drugs
— Caution is required in patients with aortic valve stenosis because of the risk of decreased perfusion of the coronary arteries caused by lowering of the blood pressure

Vasodilators
Hydralazine
The most frequently prescribed vasodilator. Its direct action on the vessels produces a reflex sympathetic response that increases heart rate and cardiac output. For this reason the drug is contraindicated in angina pectoris.

Side effects are rare and include fluid retention, headache and orthostatic hypotension.

A lupus erythematosus-like syndrome has been reported where high doses (>200 mg daily) are used. This syndrome is reversible when the drug is discontinued.

Prazosin
Prazosin is a vasodilator and alpha-blocker and dilates both the peripheral arterial and peripheral venous system, thus decreasing the blood pressure and increasing cardiac output. The drug lacks the bronchospastic effect of beta-blockers. Renal blood flow is not altered and the drug is excreted mainly in the faeces, so it can be used in renal failure provided the initial dose is reduced. Side effects include first-dose syncope, drowsiness, fluid retention and orthostatic hypotension. In patients with ischaemic heart disease prazosin may precipitate angina pectoris and therefore it should be avoided as sole therapy in these patients.

Calcium antagonists
— Verapamil is a phenylalkylamine
— Nifedipine is a dihydropyridine
— Diltiazem is a benzothiazepine
Despite their heterogeneity, these drugs are the prototypes of the rapidly expanding group of compounds known as 'calcium antagonists' or 'slow channel blockers'. Their characteristic is that they act primarily by

diminishing calcium channel activity. They differ from one another in terms of their tissue selectivity, pharmacodynamics and side effects.

— Verapamil and nifedipine dilate peripheral arteries and may be used as antihypertensive drugs
— Verapamil, nifedipine and diltiazem may be prescribed in coronary artery disease
— Verapamil may be prescribed as antiarrhythmic drug

RENOVASCULAR HYPERTENSION

This is the most frequent form of secondary hypertension in the elderly and should be suspected in the following circumstances

— If a previously normotensive patient aged 50 years or over presents with elevated blood pressure
— If blood pressure control becomes progressively difficult in a patient with essential hypertension which has been effectively controlled for several years on a stable medical regimen
— The development of severe hypertensive retinopathy or an increase in serum creatinine level should heighten suspicion of renovascular hypertension

Diagnosis

An abdominal bruit is present in approximately 50% of all patients with renovascular hypertension. In patients with evidence of generalized atherosclerotic vascular disease with bruits over the carotid, aortic, iliac and femoral areas there may be disease of the renal arteries as well.

Diagnosis of a renovascular lesion can be made by visualization of the arteries in combination with a functional assessment of the renin system at the renal vein.

Treatment

Drug therapy is the initial treatment of choice in the elderly patient with renovascular hypertension. Drug therapy alone may achieve long-term adequate blood pressure control but still not slow down the atherosclerotic disease process responsible for much of the morbidity in the elderly. During drug therapy patients must be monitored with periodic serum creatinine level and evaluation of renal size.

If blood pressure control is poor or renal function deteriorates, a different therapeutic approach should be considered. The need for surgical intervention has been diminished by the development of percutaneous transluminal angioplasty. In certain lesions, particularly ostial lesions, surgery may be required.

Nephrectomy should be considered for elderly patients with a small non-functioning kidney, with a normal contralateral kidney, uncontrolled hypertension, and differential renal vein renins showing marked lateralization to the atrophic kidney, when the uninvolved kidney is normal or hypertrophied in size and has normal arteries.

BIBLIOGRAPHY

Alderman M H, Stanback M E 1985 Hypertension. In: Exton-Smith A N, Weksler M E (eds) Practical Geriatric Medicine. Churchill Livingstone, Edinburgh. ch 25, pp 206–213

Amery A, Birkenhäger W H, Brixko P et al 1985 Mortality and morbidity results from the European Working Party on High Blood Pressure in the Elderly Trial. Lancet 1: 1349–1354

Berman N D 1983 Geriatric cardiology. Castle House, Tunbridge Wells. ch 6, pp 109–125

Birkenhäger W H, de Leeuw P W 1988 Treatment of the elderly hypertensive: A clinical perspective. In: Bexton R (ed) Risk factor modification in the elderly. European Heart Journal 9 (suppl D): 63–67

Colandrea M A, Friedman G D, Nichaman M Z, Lynd C N 1970 Systolic hypertension in the elderly: An epidemiological assessment. Circulation 41: 239–245

Dyer A R, Stamler J, Shekelle R B, Schoenberger J A, Farinaro E 1977 Hypertension in the elderly. Medical Clinics of North America 61: 513–529

Gifford R W 1982 Isolated systolic hypertension in the elderly. Some controversial issues. Journal of the American Medical Association 247: 781–785

Grobbee D E, Hofman A 1986 Does sodium restriction lower blood pressure? British Medical Journal 20: 424–426

Kannel W B 1976 Some lessons in cardiovascular epidemiology from Framingham. American Journal of Cardiology 37: 269–282

Mattila K, Haavisto M, Rajala S, Heikinheimo R 1988 Blood pressure and five year survival in the very old. British Medical Journal 1: 887–889

Messerli F H, Ventura H O, Glade L B, Sundgaard-Riisek, Dunn F G, Fromlich E D 1983 Essential hypertension in the elderly: Haemodynamics, intravascular volume, plasma renin activity and circulating catecholamine levels. Lancet 2: 983–985

Moser M 1988 Physiological differences in the elderly. Are they clinically important? In: Bexton R (ed) Risk factor modification in the elderly. European Heart Journal 9 (Suppl D): 55–61

Ostfeld A M, Shekelle R B, Tufo H M, Wieland A M, Kilbridge J A, Drori J 1971 Cardiovascular and cerebrovascular disease in an elderly poor urban population. American Journal of Public Health 61: 19–29

Rajala S, Haavisto M, Heikinheimo R, Mattila K 1983 Blood pressure and mortality in the very old. Lancet 2: 520–521

Sever P S, Fordon D, Peart W J, Beighton P 1980 Blood pressure and its correlates in urban and tribal Africa. Lancet 2: 60–64

Siersbaek-Nielsen K, Molholm Hansen J, Kampmann J, Kristensen M 1971 Rapid evaluation of creatinine clearance. Lancet 1: 1133–1134

Walsh R A 1987 Cardiovascular effects of the aging process. American Journal of Medicine 82: 34–40

Wenting G J, Tan-Tjiong H L, Derkx F H M, de Bruyn J H B, Manintveld A J, Schalekamp M A D H 1984 Split renal function after captopril in unilateral renal artery stenosis. British Medical Journal 288: 886–890

Wilkie F, Eisdorfer C 1971 Intelligence and blood pressure in the aged. Science 172: 959–962

9. HEART DISEASE

ISCHAEMIC HEART DISEASE

Ischaemia is by far the commonest cause of heart disease in old age and ischaemic heart disease is a source of significant morbidity as well as mortality.

Systemic hypertension is the most significant risk factor for the development of ischaemic heart disease in the elderly.

Glucose intolerance and the ratio of low-density lipoprotein to high-density lipoprotein cholesterol remain significant risk factors, whereas smoking and family history appear to lose their relevance after age 65.

There are three major clinical syndromes of ischaemic heart disease
— Angina pectoris (stable and unstable forms)
— Myocardial infarction
— Chronic ischaemic heart disease

ANGINA PECTORIS

Angina pectoris (angina) is pain or discomfort caused by ischaemia of the cardiac muscle. The commonest cause of angina is atherosclerosis of the coronary arteries with fixed coronary artery stenosis. However, in most patients pathophysiology is mixed and consists of a combination of fixed atherosclerosis with varying degrees of coronary artery spasm. This has implications for the medical therapy in these patients.

Clinical features

The classical symptom of angina is central chest pain or discomfort precipitated by exertion and relieved by rest. The pain is usually described as 'tight', 'heavy' or 'crushing' in nature. Radiation of the discomfort is common but extremely variable. The relationship to exertion is one of the most important aspects of angina, especially in the elderly, where a typical pressure-like sensation is often lacking. The possibility of ischaemia should be considered for any symptom, such as dyspnoea or dizziness, provoked by exertion and relieved by rest. Physical examination is often normal when the patient is at rest. Evidence of left ventricular dysfunction, i.e. a third or fourth heart sound, or signs of left ventricular failure may be present if the patient is seen immediately after an attack of angina.

The patient should be checked for hypertension, aortic valve disease, anaemia and manifestations of syphilis.

Diagnosis

The history is of paramount importance to establish the diagnosis.

Physical examination may be normal or there may be evidence of left ventricular dysfunction.

The resting electrocardiogram (ECG) may be entirely normal in the presence of severe coronary artery disease. ECG changes, particularly ST segment shifts occurring at the time of spontaneous symptoms, is diagnostic of an ischaemic basis for the symptoms.

Serum levels of intracellular enzymes are normal since angina does not cause necrosis of myocardial tissue.

Exercise testing and coronary angiography may be required to establish the diagnosis, but these are usually only done if cardiac surgery is being considered.

Management

General
— Correction of precipitating factors such as hypertension, congestive cardiac failure and anaemia should be attempted
— Regular exercise may improve exercise tolerance
— Adjustment of life-style may be required in patients with severe limitation of exertion; for some patients, this may involve moving to a more suitable home.
— Patients should be advised to reduce exertion as soon as pain occurs and to be cautious in cold weather and after a heavy meal

Specific

Nitrates
Nitrates remain the foundation of medical therapy for angina; their pharmacological action is to relax smooth muscle; the dominant effect seems to be venodilatation, as arterial vasodilatation is much less pronounced; the result is a reduction of preload and of peripheral resistance.

There is considerable variation in response to nitrate therapy amongst patients, so wide dose ranges are recommended.

Side effects are related to vasodilatation and include headache, flushing, dizziness, tachycardia and orthostatic hypotension.

Table 9.1

Product	Onset of action	Duration of action
Glyceryl trinitrate		
Sublingual tablet	2 min	20–60 min
Transdermal patch	1–2 h	24 h
Isosorbide dinitrate		
Chewable tablet	<2 min	2 h
Oral tablet	20 min	4–6 h
Isosorbide mononitrate		
Oral tablet	20–30 min	10–12 h

Patients should be advised to sit down whenever possible before taking rapid-acting nitrates.

Table 9.1 shows the action profile of the various preparations.

Preparations include
— Glyceryl trinitrate: tablets are taken sublingually to relieve angina; they are more effective if taken prior to exertion that is known to precipitate angina
— Isosorbide dinitrate: tablets may be taken regularly by mouth as a prophylaxis against angina and can be chewed for a rapid effect to relieve angina. The drug has a longer action than glyceryl trinitrate and extensive first-pass hepatic metabolism to isosorbide mononitrate occurs. High doses may be needed to obtain therapeutic systemic blood levels
— Isosorbide mononitrate: tablets can be given twice daily as a prophylaxis against angina
— No advantages have been demonstrated of topical applications of nitrates; they are expensive, can cause skin irritation and absorption is variable. Nevertheless the glyceryl trinitrate patch can be used to aid compliance (applied once daily) particularly when other routes of administration have been complicated by side effects.

Beta-blockers
If satisfactory control of symptoms cannot be achieved with nitrates alone, beta-blockers may be added provided there are no specific contraindications to their use (see also Ch. 8). A variety of beta-blockers with different ancillary properties are available and all seem to be equally effective in the treatment of angina (Thadani et al 1979).

Calcium antagonists
Nifedipine
This is a calcium antagonist and a useful prophylactic agent if coronary spasm is implicated in angina pectoris. The 10-mg capsule can be chewed and the contents held in the mouth for an immediate effect. Side effects include headache, flushing, dizziness, tachycardia and orthostatic

hypotension (see also Ch. 8). To avoid these side effects combination with a beta-blocker may be used.

Diltiazem

This is a calcium antagonist which has fewer side effects than nifedipine and can be administered as monotherapy.

Transluminal angioplasty

Experience with percutaneous transluminal coronary angioplasty in older patients is still limited. Further information regarding its usefulness in this age group is required.

Cardiac surgery

The usefulness of coronary artery (by-pass graft) surgery in older patients needs to be further evaluated.

UNSTABLE ANGINA

Unstable angina or intermediate syndrome is a syndrome intermediate between typical angina and myocardial infarction (Editorial 1980). There is a changing pattern of angina; angina occurring at rest, not provoked by emotion, is unstable, as is an increase in frequency, severity or ease of provocation of angina in a patient with previous stable angina. It may occur after a myocardial infarction.

The patient with unstable angina is at high risk of developing a myocardial infarction or sudden death, and should be admitted to hospital, preferably to a coronary care unit, for intensive medical treatment.

MYOCARDIAL INFARCTION

Myocardial infarction is the result of a sudden cessation of blood supply to part of the left ventricular myocardium with necrosis of the ischaemic tissue and eventual replacement by a fibrous scar. The commonest cause is a thrombus superimposed on an atheromatous plaque. Rarer causes include emboli originating from the left atrium or from a diseased aortic valve, or inflammatory disease of the artery. Hypotension may reduce the filling pressure of the coronary artery and precipitate a myocardial infarction in the absence of complete occlusion.

Clinical features

The *typical* presentation of myocardial infarction is a sudden severe crushing retrosternal chest pain, not related to exertion, and unrelieved by glyceryl trinitrate. The pain may radiate to the left or both shoulders and arms, into the jaw, the epigastrium or the back. Associated symptoms are sweating, faintness, nausea and vomiting. The classical

Table 9.2 Presentation of myocardial infarction

Symptom	70 (n = 125) (%)	70–74 (n = 243) (%)	Age (years) 75–79 (n = 181) (%)	80–84 (n = 140) (%)	85+ (n = 88) (%)	Total (n = 777) (%)
Chest pain	76.0	79.4	67.9	50.7	37.5	66.3
Short of breath	37.6	42.8	40.9	47.1	43.2	42.4
Syncope	8.8	8.2	14.9	21.4	18.0	13.4
Stroke	1.6	2.1	5.0	8.6	6.8	4.4
Acute confusion	3.2	2.5	8.3	7.9	19.3	6.8
Weakness	7.2	7.0	7.7	5.7	10.2	7.3
Giddiness	5.6	6.6	3.9	5.0	4.5	5.3
Palpitations	4.0	1.6	1.7	1.4	1.1	1.9
Vomiting	18.4	21.0	18.2	17.1	15.9	18.7
Sweating	36.0	32.5	27.1	17.1	13.6	26.9
Arterial embolus	0.8	0.8	–	–	–	0.4
Silent	1.6	2.1	1.8	2.8	3.3	2.2

From Bayer et al (1986).

presentation occurs in the majority of young patients with myocardial infarction, but a greater proportion of elderly patients have an *atypical* clinical picture (Pathy 1967). In a retrospective analysis of the presentation of 777 acutely ill patients aged 65–100 (mean age 76.0 years) who were admitted to geriatric medical beds during a 7-year period and who were subsequently found to have suffered an acute myocardial infarction, Bayer et al (1986) reviewed symptoms at presentation. The diagnostic criteria of Rowley & Hampton (1981) were used to indicate definite or probable myocardial infarction. Chest pain was defined as a pain, tightness, pressure or discomfort in the chest or upper abdomen. A silent myocardial infarction was said to have occurred in the absence of any symptoms but in the presence of characteristic electrocardiographic or cardiac enzyme changes on coincidental testing.

The spectrum of presentation changed significantly with increasing age (Table 9.2). Although chest pain was the most commonly reported symptom in all the elderly patients, a third did not have chest pain but presented with other symptoms. Moreover, the incidence of chest pain fell with increasing age, as did reports of sweating and vomiting. Some elderly people were unable to provide a clear history when they were confused or suffering from language or cognitive defects, psychiatric illness, or in coma. When such patients were excluded, 70% of those who did not report chest pain could be regarded as truly pain-free. Shortness of breath was the second most frequent complaint (42%), occurring in the absence of chest pain in 15%, and was equally common at all ages; in the oldest age group (85+) it replaced chest pain as the most commonly recorded symptom. Other presentations such as syncope, acute confusion and stroke were more common with increasing age and were often the sole presenting feature. Only 2% of all patients were found to have truly 'silent' myocardial infarction; the ages of these patients were equally distributed throughout the age bands examined.

Diagnosis

The diagnosis of myocardial infarction is based on the history plus the occurrence of characteristic electrocardiographic and enzyme changes (Rowley & Hampton 1981).

History and clinical features

In the absence of pain, acute shortness of breath may suggest the diagnosis, but in the elderly myocardial infarction may equally well present as cardiac failure, stroke, syncope, giddiness, weakness, acute confusion, vomiting, peripheral gangrene, or palpitations.

In some cases no abnormal physical signs are found. Transient dysrhythmias are common in the earliest stage of infarction; they carry a more serious prognosis if they persist or develop with evolution of the myocardial infarction.

Cardiogenic shock is likely to occur with damage to 40% of the myocardium. Moreover, any myocardial infarction complicated by frequent episodes of ventricular tachycardia may extend and lead to cardiogenic shock. In addition, cardiogenic shock may be initiated by acute mechanical sequelae of myocardial infarction such as major mitral valve regurgitation, ventricular septal rupture, sudden ventricular aneurysmal change or rupture in the free wall of the left ventricle with subsequent cardiac tamponade and sudden death.

In elderly patients sudden death with electromechanical dissociation is most often due to rupture of the myocardium and cardiac tamponade.

Electrocardiographic changes

Serial electrocardiograms (ECG) should be performed at least daily for the first 5 days.

- T wave change is the earliest feature: initially, T waves of increased amplitude in leads facing the site of injury may be found; later, symmetrical T wave inversion occurs
- ST segment changes occur early and consist of ST elevation in leads facing the site of injury, frequently in association with reciprocal ST depression in opposing leads
- The development of Q waves of at least 0.03 seconds or greater is perhaps the most significant, though not pathognomonic, ECG finding of an acute myocardial infarction
- In strictly posterior myocardial infarction, Q waves may be demonstrated in left posterior chest leads; the diagnosis is supported by an abnormal anterior shift in the QRS, manifested by 0.04-second R waves in leads V1 and V2.

Enzyme changes

Lactic dehydrogenase (LDH), its isoenzyme hydroxybutyrate dehydrogenase (HBD) and creatine phosphokinase (CPK) are elevated to varying levels in myocardial infarction. The MB isoenzyme of CPK is a sensitive marker of myocardial necrosis.

ESR and temperature chart

ESR and temperature chart may prove of limited value in establishing the diagnosis of myocardial infarction in the elderly.

Management

Initial acute phase

Patients with suspected myocardial infarction should be admitted to hospital, where acute thrombolysis can be carried out depending on the age of the patient and the presence of contraindications. Thrombolysis can be achieved with streptokinase or tissue plasminogen activator (TPA); TPA has the advantage of a short half-life and a short duration of action. Contraindications include: (previous) haemorrhage or predisposition to haemorrhage, for example hiatus hernia, peptic ulcer, thrombocytopenia; recent stroke (less than 3 months ago); recent trauma, for example surgery (less than 6 weeks ago).

Most deaths due to myocardial infarction occur within the first 4 hours of symptoms, and are often due to a heart rhythm disorder, especially ventricular fibrillation.

Ventricular fibrillation is the major cause of mortality in the first 24 hours of hospital admission and the only effective treatment is prompt direct current cardioversion (200–400 W/s).

Studies on the prophylactic use of lignocaine to prevent ventricular fibrillation report varying degrees of success. Evidence from various studies strongly suggests that the prophylactic dose of lignocaine most likely to significantly reduce ventricular fibrillation is critical and readily produces reversible toxic side effects. A comparison of lignocaine kinetics in six young and six elderly patients showed no difference in volume of distribution, but the half-life in the elderly was prolonged (Braunwald 1980).

Pain relief may be obtained with IV morphine, 5–10 mg, accompanied by IV administration of an antiemetic such as metoclopramide 10 mg.

The value of beta-blocking drugs to prevent recurrence of myocardial infarction in elderly patients is uncertain.

Mobilization

During the initial period of bed rest heparin should be given subcutaneously to prevent venous thromboembolism: 5000 units two to three times daily. Once pain has been relieved the patient should be encouraged to be out of bed provided there is no cardiac failure, hypotension or arrhythmia. Thereafter, activities should be increased gradually but should be limited if shortness of breath or chest pain occurs.

If early mobilization is not possible, heparin should be continued or administration of oral anticoagulants should be considered.

Complications of myocardial infarction

- Arrhythmias
- Cardiac conduction disturbances
- Cardiac failure
- Cardiogenic shock
- Pericarditis
- Mural thrombus and systemic embolism
- Left ventricular aneurysm
- Rupture of the ventricular septum or papillary muscle
- Cardiac rupture

CHRONIC ISCHAEMIC HEART DISEASE

This condition may complicate angina pectoris or myocardial infarction or may occur without a history of either condition being present. Chronic ischaemic heart disease causes cardiac failure.

CARDIAC FAILURE

Cardiac failure remains the single most common cause of death in persons over 65 years of age.

Definition

Cardiac failure is defined as the inability of the heart to pump blood adequately to meet the body's requirements.

Classification

Cardiac failure can be graded, rather imprecisely, according to the inability to exercise (Table 9.3).

Table 9.3 New York Heart Association Classification of heart failure

Class I	No limitation of physical activity
Class II	Slight limitation of physical activity
Class III	Marked limitation of physical activity
Class IV	Inability to carry out any physical activity without discomfort

Differential diagnosis

Although heart failure is not necessarily caused by myocardial failure, this is the most common mechanism, and in the elderly it is almost always a factor in heart failure of any aetiology.

Primary heart disease
Causes of cardiac failure in which the prime abnormality is an abnormality of the heart are usually associated with a low or normal cardiac output at rest, and a low cardiac output on exercise. They include:

— Myocardial disease, which may be caused by ischaemic heart disease, hypertension, alcohol, cardiomyopathy or degenerative changes
— Arrhythmias
— Disease of the cardiac valves, especially aortic valve stenosis and mitral valve stenosis or incompetence

— Drugs affecting left ventricular performance, e.g. negative inotropic effect of beta-blockers, calcium antagonists and antiarrhythmic drugs.

Secondary cardiac failure

Cardiac failure may occur secondary to other conditions, such as

— Anaemia
— Thyroid disease (both thyrotoxicosis and myxoedema)
— Extensive Paget's disease with functional arteriovenous shunt
— Chronic obstructive airways disease
— Pulmonary embolic disease

ACUTE CARDIAC FAILURE

This is a syndrome resulting from a sudden deterioration of left ventricular function. The clinical picture is one of marked breathlessness, pulmonary oedema, cyanosis and peripheral vasoconstriction. An acute cause, such as myocardial infarction or respiratory infection, is usually present, but sometimes no precipitating cause is found. These patients may have 'undulating' heart failure in which the natural history of chronic heart failure is interrupted by an episodic abrupt deterioration in myocardial function.

Clinical features of cardiac failure

Though in clinical terms one can speak of left and right heart failure, the two sides of the heart form a closed system and the stroke volume pumped from each side is essentially equal, apart from minor moment-to-moment variations.

In heart failure a compensatory increase in atrial pressures helps to maintain the cardiac output. Venoconstriction mediated by the sympathetic nervous system redistributes blood flow centrally, and activation of the renin–angiotensin system stimulates salt and water retention (Francis et al 1984).

These same neuroendocrine mechanisms increase vascular resistance, which supports the blood pressure but also creates a vicious cycle of increasing left ventricular afterload and falling cardiac output (Kluger et al 1982).

Raised atrial pressures and reduced cardiac output, expressed clinically as pulmonary and systemic congestion and peripheral hypoperfusion, cause the dyspnoea, oedema and fatigue of heart failure. Dyspnoea is worse on exertion or lying flat (both of which provoke a steep rise in the left atrial pressure) and is often accompanied by fatigue if cardiac output is inadequate for the oxygen requirement of the exercising muscle.

Central nervous system symptoms such as confusion, memory

Table 9.4 Physical signs associated with heart failure

Dyspnoea, orthopnoea, pulmonary oedema
Tachycardia
Elevated jugular venous pressure more than 3 cm above the sternal angle
Hepatomegaly
Oedema in the dependent parts of the body (e.g. oedema over the sacrum in bed-bound patients)
Peripheral vasoconstriction

Additional signs
Pleural effusions (can occur with failure of either ventricle)
Ascites(can occur in long-standing chronic congestive cardiac failure, tricuspid valve incompetence, constrictive pericarditis)
Cheyne–Stokes respiration (can occur due to low cardiac output)
Cardiac enlargement (heart size may be normal in patients with constrictive pericarditis and acute heart failure)
A third and/or fourth heart sound* (can occur due to failure of the ventricules; a third heart sound in an elderly person is always abnormal and indicative of left ventricular failure)
Presence of a systolic regurgitation murmur*

*The third heart sound and the systolic regurgitation murmur may disappear with treatment of heart failure.

impairment and insomnia may occur due to low cardiac output.

The physical signs of heart failure are listed in Table 9.4.

Investigations

— Chest X-ray
— Electrocardiogram
— Full blood count
— Urea and electrolytes
— Serum creatinine level
— Cardiac enzymes

Optional investigations

— Thyroid function tests (often indicated even in the absence of clinical features of thyroid disease)
— Echocardiography (on indication)
— Cardiac catheterization (should be performed when there is major diagnostic doubt or when a condition amenable to surgery is suspected)

Management

Identification and correction of the cause of heart failure should be attempted. Aggravating factors, particularly arrhythmias and hypertension, should also be corrected. Patients should be advised to maintain an optimal weight, to avoid excessive intake of salt and alcohol, and to stop smoking.

Further treatment is aimed at controlling symptoms and slowing the progression of the disease by lowering atrial pressures and improving cardiac output.

In *acute heart failure* with pulmonary oedema the patient should be allowed to sit up and oxygen should be administered; blood gas analysis is necessary during the initial phase. Morphine acts centrally to reduce anxiety and diminish reflex sympathetic activation, thus having a vasodilator effect. The elderly are particularly prone to the respiratory depression and hypotensive effects of morphine, so initially small doses should be administered IV so that the peak effect can be anticipated in 15–20 minutes and observed. Frusemide relieves symptoms before any diuretic effect occurs, probably by acting as a vasodilator. IV morphine 5–10 mg, or IV diamorphine 5 mg, is given slowly over 3–5 minutes, together with IV frusemide, 40–80 mg. If the diagnosis is doubtful and asthma or respiratory disease is the alternative diagnosis, morphine is contraindicated because it is a respiratory depressant, and IV aminophylline should be given. Digoxin has no place in the immediate treatment of acute heart failure.

In *chronic heart failure* diuretics are the drugs of first choice, and often no other treatment is necessary. They promote excretion of salt and water, reducing the plasma volume and atrial pressures. Over-use of diuretics must be avoided since reduction of preload may result in a reduction of cardiac output. Especially in elderly patients with so-called 'stiff left ventricle' there is a delicate balance between signs of congestive heart failure and signs of low circulating blood volume, e.g. due to dehydration. Therefore, the use of diuretics should be carefully monitored. If patients require more than 40 mg a day of frusemide (or its equivalent) a low dose of an angiotensin converting enzyme (ACE) inhibitor, such as captopril 12.5 mg or enalapril 2.5 mg twice daily, should be added. The dose may be increased if blood pressure and renal function remain satisfactory. Although conventional vasodilators such as nitrates, prazosin and hydralazine reduce atrial pressures and improve cardiac output, tolerance is common and the capacity for exercise rarely improves. Therefore, they are less effective than ACE inhibitors for treating heart failure and are now rarely used (Bayliss et al 1985).

The inotropic effect of digitalis improves cardiac output, but in sinus rhythm the responses are minimal and the narrow therapeutic range makes the ratio of risk to benefit too high for most patients. In addition, the impaired renal function which is found with severe heart failure calls for careful dose monitoring. It remains the best drug for controlling heart rate in atrial fibrillation in the presence or absence of heart failure.

DISORDERS OF CARDIAC RHYTHM AND CONDUCTION

Disorders of cardiac rhythm and conduction are very common in elderly people. The cardiac dysrhythmias may be classified by site and duration; they may be supraventricular, atrioventricular or ventricular (Tables 9.5 and 9.6); they may be either brief, involving one to five beats,

Table 9.5 Prevalence (%) of tachyarrhythmia in 1171 institutionalized elderly people

Sick sinus syndrome	0.3
Supraventricular tachycardia	2.5
Atrial flutter	1.8
Atrial fibrillation	14.7
Ventricular tachycardia	0.1
Ventricular fibrillation	0.2

From Caird (1985)

Table 9.6 Prevalence (%) of conduction disorders in the elderly

	General elderly population	Institutionalized elderly
1° atrioventricular block	1	2–10
2° atrioventricular block		1–2
3° atrioventricular block		0.2–0.9
RBBB	2–3.5	4–13
LBBB	0.6–2.5	4–5.7
LAH ('Left anterior hemiblock')	2	6–27
RBBB + LAH	1	0.5–9

From Caird (1985).

paroxysmal or sustained; they may occur with myocardial infarction or thyrotoxicosis.

Syncope of the Stokes–Adams type is characterized by sudden onset, occurrence of pallor at onset and flushing on recovery, and an absent or very slow pulse during the attack.

ATRIAL FIBRILLATION

This is the most common paroxysmal and persistent arrhythmia in the elderly and is often associated with heart disease, particularly ischaemic, hypertensive, valvular, alcoholic and thyrotoxic heart disease; it may occur with infections and with cardiac involvement in malignant disease.

In the elderly, atrial fibrillation is commonly present with a controlled ventricular response rate; if this is a stable situation, no therapy is required. Atrial fibrillation with a high ventricular response rate should be treated with digitalization, aiming at a ventricular rate of 60–70 beats/min at rest.

Digoxin has a low therapeutic index and is excreted almost completely unchanged by the kidneys (see also Ch. 30). Therefore, excretion may be impaired when renal function deteriorates from normal. Hypokalaemia and hypomagnesaemia increase the sensitivity to digoxin. Monitoring of serum digoxin levels, renal function and electrolyte status is required for elderly patients on digoxin.

The combination of digoxin and a beta-blocker may improve control of ventricular rate, especially during exercise.

Aspirin (300 mg daily) may be given in order to prevent thromboembolism in patients with atrial fibrillation who have had one or more transient ischaemic attacks (see Ch. 3).

PAROXYSMAL ATRIAL FIBRILLATION

If conversion to sinus rhythm is necessary, elective direct current cardioversion is the procedure of choice. If the left atrium is enlarged, heparinization or anticoagulation should be started 3–5 days prior to cardioversion, since the risk of systemic embolism is highest at restoration of sinus rhythm with cardioversion; anticoagulation should be continued for 3 months after restoration of sinus rhythm, provided there are no contraindications, because of the high risk of systemic embolism at recurrence of atrial fibrillation.

Disopyramide (50 mg) can be given IV 30 minutes before cardioversion; quinidine is an alternative choice.

If sinus rhythm is obtained the patient is continued on digoxin or verapamil in order to prevent recurrence of atrial fibrillation; if cardioversion is unsuccessful the patient may be continued on digoxin in order to control ventricular response rate, if necessary.

PACEMAKER THERAPY

Symptomatic third-degree (complete) atrioventricular block is an indication for pacing. If a patient with sick sinus syndrome and tachycardia cannot be managed with medical treatment, pacemaker therapy is needed.

The combination of right bundle branch block with left anterior hemiblock (bifascicular block) is not an indication for pacing, since the prognosis is no different from right bundle branch block alone; pacing should be confined to patients with documented symptomatic arrhythmias (McAnulty et al 1978).

VALVULAR HEART DISEASE

Aortic valve disease

Aortic valve stenosis
Calcification of a congenitally bicuspid valve is the most common cause of isolated aortic valve stenosis, but the frequency of this pathological finding decreases with increasing age.

After age 75 degenerative calcification of normal valves accounts for almost all cases of isolated aortic valve stenosis. The rate of progression of stenosis is variable and independent of the cause of stenosis. Associated aortic valve incompetence can be found in about 50% of patients with aortic valve stenosis.

Aortic valve incompetence
This is the most common valve lesion in the elderly. About 40% of patients with rheumatic mitral valve disease and about 50% of patients with aortic valve stenosis of any aetiology have associated aortic valve incompetence.

Mitral valve disease

Mitral valve stenosis in the elderly is almost always rheumatic in origin. The prevalence of rheumatic mitral valve disease in the elderly is estimated at 2–3%; in one-third stenosis predominates, while in the remainder incompetence is the dominant lesion. Mitral valve stenosis may be mimicked by calcification of the mitral annulus or by left atrial myxoma. Mitral valve incompetence may result from papillar muscle dysfunction secondary to coronary artery disease, left ventricular enlargement of any origin, or mitral valve prolapse.

Systemic emboli occur in about 6% of elderly patients with predominant mitral valve stenosis, but are uncommon in elderly patients with predominant mitral valve incompetence.

In elderly patients, mitral valve disease is almost always associated with atrial fibrillation and therefore anticoagulation is warranted in these patients. If anticoagulants are contraindicated aspirin may be considered.

Tricuspid valve disease

Tricuspid valve stenosis is rare in the elderly. Tricuspid valve incompetence is relatively common and is usually secondary to right ventricular failure.

Multivalvular disease

In the elderly multivalvular disease usually consists of a combination of mitral and aortic valve disease, in which the disease of one valve predominates and the therapeutic approach should be the same as for the dominant lesion in isolation.

INFECTIVE ENDOCARDITIS

This condition has a high mortality of approximately 30% in elderly patients — twice that in younger patients (Wedgwood 1976). The diagnosis is often delayed in the elderly, partly because it is often not clinically suspected at all for the following reasons:
— There is a mistaken impression that endocarditis is rare in old age
— Less than one-third of elderly patients present with typical features and even these tend to be modified in the older age group
— The presence of other pathological processes obscures the diagnosis

Predisposing factors are underlying rheumatic heart disease (especially rheumatic mitral valve incompetence), non-rheumatic cardiac abnormalities (especially those involving the aortic valve), mitral valve prolapse, calcification of the mitral annulus and the presence of prosthetic valves. In approximately one-third of patients no underlying heart disease can be found (Thell et al 1975). The condition is characterized by the combination of fever and heart murmur, but both may be absent. In the elderly, basal body temperature is generally lower, and unless this is taken into consideration a low-grade fever is apt to be missed. Heart murmurs are often soft, and by themselves are not likely to arouse suspicion, as such murmurs are common in the elderly. Congestive cardiac failure may be present. Atrial fibrillation is not uncommon. Splenomegaly is present in about one-third of cases, petechiae and splinter haemorrhages in about 10% of cases or less, and clubbing, Osler's nodes, Roth spots and Janeway lesions are even less common (Berman 1983). Two-dimensional echocardiography is a very sensitive technique for detecting vegetations on the valves, particularly aortic and tricuspid vegetations, and has been positive in up to 80% of patients with endocarditis (Melvin et al 1981). Blood cultures are the most critical of the laboratory tests. Other frequent features are a raised ESR, anaemia, reduction in platelet count, hyperglobulinaemia, presence of rheumatoid factor and microscopic haematuria.

The treatment of endocarditis consists of IV administration of antibiotics for minimally 4 weeks followed by oral therapy for the latter part of the course of treatment. The choice of antibiotic depends on the responsible organism and its sensitivity.

If haemodynamic deterioration occurs cardiac surgery can be a life-saving procedure in selected patients.

BIBLIOGRAPHY

Bayer A J, Chadha J S, Farag R R, Pathy M S J 1986 Changing presentation of myocardial infarction with increasing age. Journal of the American Geriatrics Society 34: 263–266

Bayliss R I S 1985 The silent coronary. British Medical Journal 290: 1093–1094

Bayliss J, Norell M S, Canepa-Anson R, Reid C, Poole-Wilson P, Sutton G 1985 Clinical importance of the renin–angiotensin system in chronic heart failure: Double blind comparison of captopril and prazosin. British Medical Journal 290: 1861–1866

Berman N D (ed) 1983 Infective endocarditis. In: Geriatric cardiology. Castle House, Tunbridge Wells. ch 7, pp 133–136

Braunwald E 1980 Treatment of the patient after myocardial infarction: The last decade and the next. New England Journal of Medicine 302: 290–293

Caird F I 1985 Disorders of cardiac rhythm and conduction. In: Exton-Smith A N, Weksler M E (eds) Practical Geriatric Medicine. Churchill Livingstone, Edinburgh, p. 202

Editorial 1980 Unstable angina. Lancet 2: 569–570

Francis G S, Goldsmith S R, Levine T B, Olivari M T, Cohn J N 1984 The neurohumeral axis in congestive heart failure. Annals of Internal Medicine 101: 370–377

Kluger J, Cody R J, Laragh J H 1982 The contributions of sympathetic tone and the renin–angiotensin system to severe chronic congestive heart failure: Response to specific inhibitors (prazosin and captopril). American Journal of Cardiology 49: 1667–1674

Levy R A, Charuzi Y, Mandell W J 1977 Lignocaine: A new technique for intravenous administration. British Heart Journal 39: 1026–1028

McAnulty J H, Rahimtoolah S H, Murphy E S et al 1978 A prospective study of sudden death in high-risk bundle branch block. New England Journal of Medicine 299: 209–215

Melvin E T, Berger M, Lutzker L G, Goldberg E, Mildvan D 1981 Non-invasive methods for detection of valve vegetations in infective endocarditis. American Journal of Cardiology 47: 271–278

Murphy P J, Van der Cammen T J M, Malone-Lee J 1986 Captopril in elderly patients with heart failure. British Medical Journal 293: 239–240

Pathy M S 1967 Clinical presentation of myocardial infarction in the elderly. British Heart Journal 29: 190–199

Rowley J M, Hampton J R 1981 Diagnostic criteria for myocardial infarction. British Journal of Hospital Medicine 26: 253–258

Stout R W 1985 Cardiovascular disease, atherosclerosis and ischaemic heart disease. In Exton-Smith A N, Weksler M E (eds) Practical Geriatric Medicine. Churchill Livingstone, Edinburgh. ch 22, pp 182–190

Thadani U, Davidson C, Singleton W, Taylor S H 1979 Comparison of the immediate effects of five beta-adrenoceptor-blocking drugs with different ancillary properties in angina pectoris. New England Journal of Medicine 300: 750–755

Thell R, Martin F H, Edwards J E 1975 Bacterial endocarditis in subjects 60 years of age and older. Circulation 51: 174–182

Timmis A D 1988 Modern treatment of heart failure. British Medical Journal 297: 83–84.

Timmis A J 1987 The third heart sound. British Medical Journal 294: 326–327

Wedgwood J 1976 Remediable heart disease. In: Caird F I, Dalt J L C, Kennedy R D (eds) Cardiology in old age. Plenum Press, New York. p 249

10. ORTHOSTATIC HYPOTENSION AND SYNCOPE

ORTHOSTATIC HYPOTENSION

Definition

Orthostatic hypotension (OH) is arbitrarily defined as a fall in systolic pressure of 20 mmHg or more on standing for 1–2 minutes. The more profound the fall in pressure the greater is its clinical significance.

Normal regulation of arterial pressure

Normally on standing after lying supine, sympathetic activity increases, causing constriction of the arterioles and veins, and parasympathetic activity decreases, causing cardiac acceleration. This change in posture produces large volume shifts and about 700 ml of blood leaves the chest and is rapidly pooled in the venous reservoirs of the abdomen and leg. Pressure in the right atrium falls to or below the intrathoracic pressure and the return of blood to the right side of the heart is reduced. Stroke volume is decreased and consequently blood pressure falls. In a fit young adult systemic arterial pressure drops only transiently on standing and within 15–30 seconds the pressure returns to the previous level or slightly above this.

Pathophysiology

In old people homeostasis is less well maintained and a change from the lying to the upright position is often accompanied by a fall in systemic blood pressure. Apart from the clinical factors, which are considered later, the decline in efficiency of homeostatic regulation with age is probably due to:

— A diminished functional capacity of the autonomic nervous system
— Age-related changes in the vascular tree with loss of elasticity in the arterial wall

Prevalence

In a study in Glasgow of people over the age of 65 living at home, systolic pressure on standing fell by:
— 20 mmHg or more in 24%
— 30 mmHg or more in 9%
— 40 mmHg or more in 5%
There was little difference in prevalence between the sexes, but it increased with age; a fall in systolic pressure of 20 mmHg or more occurred in 16% of those aged 65–74 years and in 30% of those aged over 75 years.

Two or more of the following factors — varicose veins, urinary tract infection, absent ankle jerks, anaemia, hyponatraemia, and the use of potentially hypotensive drugs — were found in 50% of subjects with a fall in systolic pressure of 30 mmHg or more but in only 17% without OH.

An even higher frequency of OH is found in patients in institutions. This has been attributed to illness and to the effects of prolonged recumbency (see below).

Aetiology

In any one patient there are often several factors leading to OH:
— Age-related decline in the function of the autonomic nervous system and possibly loss of elasticity in the arterial wall
— Impairment of baro-reflex activity due to prolonged bed rest. The effect of physical inactivity is particularly seen in elderly patients who have suffered a myocardial infarction and in whom blood pressure is maintained by near-maximal vasoconstriction. On assuming the upright posture there are too few reserves to call upon and blood pressure falls
— Hypovolaemia and hyponatraemia due to a variety of causes, including the use of thiazide and other diuretics, and in some patients an impairment of autonomic function. Excessive loss of sodium and water occurs in these patients when they are recumbent at night
— Drugs with hypotensive actions. Some of these which are commonly prescribed in the elderly are
  • Thiazides and other diuretics
  • Phenothiazines
  • Tricyclic antidepressants
  • Butyrophenones
  • Levodopa
  • Bromocriptine

Table 10.1 Diseases affecting the autonomic nervous system

Central	Autonomic neuropathy
Parkinsonism	Diabetes mellitus
Shy–Drager Syndrome	Malignancy
Wernicke's encephalopathy	Amyloidosis
Hypothalamic lesions	Acute infective polyneuropathy
Cerebrovascular disease	(Guillain–Barré syndrome)
Tabes dorsalis	Vitamin B complex deficiency
Paraplegia	Chronic alcoholism

— Diuretics reduce circulatory blood volume, whereas others such as the phenothiazines impair autonomic function.
— Diseases affecting autonomic function. Some of the more important diseases which can cause central disturbances and peripheral damage (autonomic neuropathy) are shown in Table 10.1

OH, together with other manifestations of autonomic dysfunction, can occur in all these conditions.

Parkinsonism

Tests of autonomic function, including the investigation of blood pressure control, should be made in all patients suffering from parkinsonism. The resting blood pressure is often lower than would be expected for the patient's age. Levodopa therapy sometimes first reveals evidence of autonomic dysfunction. Some of the patients with parkinsonism have the Shy–Drager syndrome, in which the somatic symptoms precede the dysautonomia.

Shy–Drager syndrome

This is a rare condition in which all the features of autonomic dysfunction are present, including profound fall in blood pressure on standing. The somatic manifestations, which include unsteadiness of gait, rigidity of the limbs, tremor and other features of parkinsonism, can appear after an interval of 6 months to 20 years.

Wernicke's encephalopathy

This condition is due to thiamine deficiency often associated with alcoholism. Characteristic petechial haemorrhages are found in the walls of the third ventricle, the hypothalamus and mamillary bodies. In one series OH was present in 80% of the patients. Other features include ophthalmoplegia, nystagmus, Korsakoff's psychosis, ataxia, peripheral neuropathy and hypothermia.

Cerebrovascular disease

OH has been attributed to cerebrovascular disease, especially in elderly hospital patients. It is possible, however, that the debility caused by the disease is a more important factor. The use of psychotropic drugs is a contributory factor in some cases.

Autonomic neuropathy

Diabetes mellitus is the commonest cause. Manifestations include dizziness and faintness due to postural falls in blood pressure, intermittent nocturnal diarrhoea, gastric fullness, dysuria and impaired temperature regulation. Elderly diabetic patients in whom urodynamic investigation reveals a hypotonic bladder should have further tests of autonomic function. The presence of autonomic impairment in diabetes carries a poor prognosis.

Clinical features

— OH is often asymptomatic even with falls in systolic pressure as great as 30 mmHg. In these cases autoregulation of the cerebral circulation, which is usually maintained in old age, is able to compensate for the fall in arterial pressure
— When compensatory mechanisms fail the patient complains of weakness, faintness, dizziness, loss of balance and blacking out when rising from the lying position
— A fall due to OH may be responsible for a fracture or hypothermia when the patient is living in cold conditions
— Other manifestations of autonomic dysfunction may be present, such as sweating abnormalities, pupillary changes, gastrointestinal disturbances, bladder dysfunction and nocturnal polyuria
— A post-prandial reduction in blood pressure has been reported by Lipsitz & Fullerton (1986) in apparently healthy elderly people. The fall in blood pressure was significantly greater than that occurring in young control subjects. The mechanism is not fully understood but it is likely that the pooling of splanchnic blood reduces the return of venous blood to the heart. It is also possible that insulin release following a meal may impair insulin-mediated sympathetic nervous system activation

Investigations

The diagnosis is established by measuring the blood pressure in the lying and standing position and finding that the systolic pressure falls by 20 mmHg or more.

On the basis of a full history and clinical examination it should be ascertained if any of the causes in Table 10.1 are present.

Many tests of autonomic function are unsuitable for the elderly. Collins et al (1980) have described more appropriate tests, described below.

Heart-rate response to standing

In young adults an increase of about 20 beats/min occurs, whereas in middle and old age it is only about 10–15 beats/min. The R–R interval on the ECG has been shown to be the shortest usually at the 15th beat

after standing in young adults, followed by a maximum increase at the
30th beat (Ewing et al 1978). This '30 : 15 ratio' is similar in normal
elderly, although the response may be flattened. In diabetic patients with
autonomic neuropathy the response is absent.

Vasomotor thermoregulatory function

Peripheral blood flow can be measured during a cycle of neutral, cool
and warm environments using a specially designed air-conditioned bed.
A poor vasoconstrictor response on cooling is found in about one-third
of healthy elderly people. The response is even further reduced by
diseases affecting the autonomic nervous system. The test is valuable in
the investigation of autonomic function in patients who have suffered
from hypothermia; there is a significant relationship between poor
thermoregulatory responsiveness and the presence of OH.

Lower body negative pressure (LBNP)

Application of negative pressure to the lower body causes pooling of
blood in the legs, increase in heart rate, decreased systolic and mean
blood pressure, reduction in peripheral blood flow and decreased cardiac
output. Reduction in systolic pressure and in heart rate occurs earlier
and at smaller imposed negative pressure in the elderly compared with
the young. Moreover, a given fall in systolic pressure in the elderly is
accompanied by a much smaller increment in heart rate.

Patients with widespread autonomic dysfunction may show negligible
changes in heart rate, but the blood pressure falls precipitously on
LBNP. The test is well tolerated by elderly people and it avoids the
practical difficulties inherent in postural tests on relatively immobile
older patients.

Management

General measures

Head-up tilt at night is considered by Bannister (1988) to be the first
line of treatment. This procedure has been shown to increase the
patient's blood volume by reducing the nocturnal water and sodium loss.
When the patient is maintained in the head-up tilt position the body
weight can increase by several kilograms. If, however, the patient
resumes the lying-flat position the circulatory blood volume decreases
and the nocturnal water and sodium loss recurs.

Any correctable cause of OH should be treated and drugs with
potentially hypotensive action should be withdrawn.

Specific measures

There have been many approaches to the management of OH but none
has proved entirely satisfactory:

      — Antigravity measures: pooling of blood on assuming the
          upright position may be prevented by mechanical means, for
          example, by wearing an anti-gravity suit, but this is not
          usually practical in the elderly. Elastic stockings to be

effective have to be full-length and used in combination with an elastic abdominal support

— Expansion of blood volume: the mineralocorticoid hormone fludrocortisone can be effective in moderate OH. The starting dose should be small (0.1 mg) and increased to a maximum of 1.0 mg daily. With large doses there is a risk of supine hypertension and the development of cardiac failure and pulmonary oedema

— Vasoconstrictor agents. Several of these have been tried
  • Flurbiprofen, a prostaglandin synthetase inhibitor, in a dose of 50 mg daily, combined with fludrocortisone
  • Pindolol is used for its sympathomimetic action in a dose of 15 mg daily. The earlier reports of its effectiveness need to be confirmed
  • Dihydroergotamine (DHE) has a vasoconstrictor action on the capacity vessels of the venous reservoirs. The usual dose is 2 mg three times daily, but the bioavailability when given orally is low
  • Midodrine, a new adrenergic agonist, (2.5–5.0 mg three times a day). Significant improvement has been reported by Schirger et al (1981) in a small series of patients with severe OH

— In postprandial hypotension caffeine has been shown to prevent the fall of blood pressure in patients with autonomic failure. This occurs on a single occasion (caffeine 200–250 mg) or when the treatment is continued over a period of 7 days. This dose of caffeine can be provided by two cups of coffee

SYNCOPE

Definition

Syncope is a transient loss of consciousness due to failure to maintain an adequate cerebral blood flow. In old age the cerebral circulation less easily adapts to a fall in arterial blood pressure owing to impairment of autoregulation.

Aetiology

Syncope can be due to a fall in cardiac output, a decrease in peripheral resistance or to local abnormality of blood vessels supplying the brain.

Cardiac syncope
Bradycardia is an important cause of cardiac syncope which occurs especially in patients with second-degree heart block when the block is

irregular, leading to periods of prolonged asystole. When the heart rate is extremely slow, complete heart block may present with Stokes–Adams attacks, in which the patient loses consciousness and falls to the ground.

Tachycardia, associated with paroxysmal dysrhythmias, may produce syncope; owing to the abbreviated diastole the filling of the heart is inadequate and output falls.

In the elderly an important cause is the sick sinus syndrome, which is characterized by chaotic atrial activity.

Syncope also occurs in cardiac infarction, angina, aortic stenosis, aortic incompetence, mitral stenosis and in ball-valve thrombus of the mitral valve.

Vasovagal syncope

This is less common in the elderly than in the young. The attack may be precipitated by standing in a crowded place, by anxiety, pain and emotional stress. Bradycardia is due to excessive vagal tone and there is a fall in peripheral resistance due to vasodilatation in the muscles.

Carotid sinus syncope

Hypersensitivity of the carotid sinus can give rise to extreme sinus bradycardia or asystole. It occurs especially in older men and may be associated with the wearing of a tight collar.

Cough syncope

Repeated coughing can lead to syncope. This is believed to result from a diminution in venous return due to a rise in intrathoracic pressure or to stimulation of baroreceptor reflexes by pressure transients occurring during coughing.

Micturition syncope

This condition occurs when blood pressure falls suddenly following decompression of a chronically distended bladder. It is probable that the combination of OH and inhibitory impulses from the bladder is of greater importance than OH alone. Fatigue, alcohol, previous sleep loss and relative fasting appear to be predisposing factors. Micturition syncope tends to occur early in the morning when the vasodilatation and low blood pressure are most marked.

Defaecation syncope

Pathy (1978) has described nine patients with a clearly defined history of syncope occurring immediately after, but sometimes during, the act of defaecation. It is probably at least as common or even more common than micturition syncope. The mechanism is believed to be similar. Syncope has been recorded following digital rectal examination, sigmoidoscopy, following manual evacuation of faeces and during barium enema examination.

Clinical features

The characteristic symptoms occurring during a syncopal attack are dizziness, nausea, visual disturbances, pallor and loss of consciousness. If the patient remains in the recumbent position consciousness may be regained within a few minutes, but the syncope can recur if the patient stands up too quickly. Recurrence is very likely if the cause is hypotension associated with cardiac infarction. Convulsions sometimes occur after the loss of consciousness, but when they come first the diagnosis is more likely to be epilepsy.

Diagnosis

— When dysrhythmias are suspected to be the cause of syncope ambulant electrocardiographic monitoring should be carried out. Episodic ECG abnormalities are frequently found in older people, but the difficulty is to relate them to syncopal attacks since they often occur during periods of freedom from clinical events. Equally the patient may activate the clinical event button on the monitor when the tracing shows no disturbance. A causal relationship is more readily established when successful treatment of the dysrhythmia leads to cessation of the syncopal attacks

— Establishing the cause of syncope in the elderly is not always straightforward, owing to difficulty in obtaining an accurate history. If possible a description of the attack should be obtained from a witness

— In transient ischaemic attacks loss of consciousness, if it occurs, is usually associated with focal neurological signs (see Ch. 3)

— Consciousness is either not lost or only momentarily lost in drop attacks (see Ch. 25)

— The diagnosis of carotid sinus syncope can often be confirmed by carotid sinus compression using continuous electrocardiographic monitoring. This must be carried out cautiously using pressure on only one side at a time

Management

It is especially important to prevent syncopal attacks in old people since falls may have serious consequences, such as fractures and hypothermia. The management of OH has already been discussed; if the patient is having hypotensive agents the dose should be reduced gradually since their sudden withdrawal in patients who were hypertensive prior to treatment may lead to cerebral haemorrhage.

Post-micturition syncope occurs almost entirely in men. It can be prevented by adopting the sitting position for micturition.

The treatment of dysrhythmias leading to cardiac syncope, including the indications for the insertion of a pacemaker, is discussed in Ch. 9. The introduction of a pacemaker is also probably the treatment of choice in patients with carotid sinus hypersensitivity.

BIBLIOGRAPHY

Bannister R (ed) 1988 Autonomic failure. Oxford University Press, Oxford

Collins K J, Exton-Smith A N, James W H, Oliver D J 1980 Functional changes in autonomic nervous responses with ageing. Age and Ageing 9: 17–24

Ewing D J, Campbell I W, Murray A, Neilson J M M, Clake B F 1978 Immediate heart rate responses to standing: Simple test for autonomic neuropathy in diabetes. British Medical Journal 1: 145–147

Lipsitz L A, Fullerton K J 1986 Postprandial blood pressure reduction in healthy elderly. Journal of American Geriatrics Society 34: 267–270

Pathy M S 1978 Defaecation syncope. Age and Ageing 7: 233–236

Schirger A, Sheps S G, Thomas J E, Fealey R D 1981 Midodrine: A new agent in the management of idiopathic orthostatic hypotension and Shy–Drager syndrome. Mayo Clinic Proceedings 56: 429–433

11. RESPIRATORY DISEASE

AGE-RELATED CHANGES

With increasing age, the alveolar walls thicken, there is a fall in the number of capillaries, increase in size of alveoli, increase in thickness of elastic fibres around the alveolar ducts, increase in size of mucous glands and calcification of cartilage. In addition, there is increased kyphosis and increased rigidity of the chest wall, which interferes with respiration. The effect of these changes is to lead to a fall in elastic recoil, in forced vital capacity and in expiratory volume in one second, and an increase in residual volume. Clinically, these changes lead to breathlessness on exertion.

PNEUMONIA

— Pneumonia is defined as inflammation of the lungs caused by microorganisms, which could be bacteria, fungi or viruses
— Bacterial pneumonia may be confined to a single lobe (lobar pneumonia), though in the elderly it is often more patchy and widespread (bronchopneumonia) with a few focal clinical signs and little obvious shadowing on chest X-ray
— The condition is common in older people, particularly those with neurological disorders (e.g. Parkinson's disease or cerebrovascular accident), those with difficulty in swallowing and with chest deformity, patients with rheumatoid disease, alcoholism and heart failure, and the elderly with previous lung disease. The classical features, such as fever, cough, pleuritic pain and breathlessness, are less common, and instead an elderly person may present with a fall or confusion. The other factor which makes the diagnosis difficult is the common occurrence of crepitations in old people, particularly in those lying in bed or with pre-existing chronic airflow obstruction

Management

Treatment is with antibiotics for the offending organism.

— Pneumonia complicating chronic airflow obstruction is usually due to pneumococcus (*Streptococcus pneumoniae*) or *Haemophilus influenzae*. The organisms are usually sensitive to a variety of antibiotics, including ampicillin, co-trimoxazole, cephalosporins, as well as tetracyclines

— Lobar pneumonia in an elderly person is more likely to be due to pneumococcal infection, although atypical organisms such as *Mycoplasma* or *Legionella* may produce a similar clinical picture. Benzylpenicillin is the drug of choice for pneumococcal infection. If the patient is hypersensitive to penicillin then erythromycin or rifampicin may be used. Erythromycin, of course, will also cover atypical organisms such as *Mycoplasma* or *Legionella*

— Aspiration pneumonia is also common in the elderly, particularly those with neurological disease and those with severe gastro-oesophageal reflux. Pneumonitis is not only due to the inflammation caused by the gastric contents, but also to the gastric flora, which may contain coliforms, staphylococci and anaerobes. Metronidazole should be used if aspiration of stomach contents is suspected, together with flucloxacillin and a broad-spectrum antibiotic

— Staphylococcal pneumonia is common, particularly during influenza epidemics. The illness is usually serious and can lead to abscess formation. Treatment should include at least two antibiotics to which the organism is sensitive, e.g. flucloxacillin and erythromycin

— In addition to antibiotic therapy, it is important that the patient is given oxygen if he or she is hypoxic, fluid to treat as well as prevent dehydration and inhaled bronchodilators to treat the associated bronchospasm and to encourage mucociliary clearance of sputum

— If, despite adequate treatment, the patient fails to respond, then one must consider either that the organism is not sensitive to the antibiotic being used or the patient has developed complications of pneumonia, which may include an abscess or empyema

TUBERCULOSIS

Although the incidence of tuberculosis has declined dramatically, it remains an important problem, particularly in the elderly. Since 1966, the highest age-related notification rate in males has been in the 60+ age group.

Presentation

The disease may present as reactivation of pulmonary lesions in the upper lobes, as pleural effusion, with lymph node involvement (particularly common in elderly men), or cryptic miliary tuberculosis. The symptoms and signs in the majority of patients are similar to those in younger patients, although the presentation of cryptic miliary tuberculosis is much more common in the elderly than in younger patients. The features of the latter include weight loss, anaemia, mild abnormality of liver function tests and pyrexia. As the chest X-ray in these patients is often normal, they are diagnosed as having malignancy, and sometimes the diagnosis of tuberculosis is only confirmed at autopsy.

Management

— Once diagnosis of tuberculosis is made, the patient should be investigated thoroughly to obtain microbiological proof of the diagnosis; but if the patient is ill, antituberculous therapy should be initiated

— Investigations which should be carried out to confirm the diagnosis include sputum staining and culture for acid-fast bacillae, gastric washings for culture, transbronchial biopsy in those with suspected diffuse disease, and liver and bone marrow biopsy for staining and culture. Tuberculin test in the elderly, unfortunately, can produce misleading results as it can be negative in those with miliary tuberculosis, in those with other infections, patients on steroid therapy, with poor nutritional status, in chronic renal failure, and elderly with lymphoma

— The recommended regimen of treatment consists of using rifampicin, isoniazid, pyrazinamide and ethambutol or streptomycin for 6 months. After 2 months, if the organism

Table 11.1 Adverse reactions of antituberculous drugs

Drug	Adverse effects
Rifampicin	Nausea, vomiting, anorexia Abnormal liver function test Hepatitis Allergic rash
Isoniazid	Peripheral neuropathy Hepatitis Muscle pain, 'frozen shoulder' Arthropathy, restlessness Insomnia, loss of memory
Pyrazinamide	Arthralgia Hepatitis
Ethambutol	Optic neuritis
Streptomycin	Ototoxicity

is sensitive to rifampicin and isoniazid, ethambutol and pyrazinamide are stopped
— Adverse reactions due to antituberculous drugs are said to be more common in the elderly and include those listed in the Table 11.1
— Prognosis in the elderly is poor. Mortality rate is high, but this reflects the high incidence of other diseases in the elderly

ASTHMA

— Asthma can be defined as the variable obstruction of intrapulmonary airways, which can be worse in the morning or after effort, and which responds to specific medication. Although it can begin at any age its prevalence in the elderly is about 6.5%. Diagnosis is often difficult and may be missed because
  • Patients may also have symptoms of chronic bronchitis
  • There may be a lack of evidence of atopy
  • It is not appreciated that asthma can occur in the elderly
— Wheezing may not be an obvious feature and the patient may instead have a cough or breathlessness. These symptoms classically occur at night time
— If the symptoms are unspecific, objective tests should be carried out to confirm the diagnosis; these include demonstration of 20% increase in the peak expiratory flow rate, following administration of a bronchodilator

Treatment

— Although asthma can present with mild attacks, it is a potentially fatal condition and this has to be appreciated not only by patients but also by the doctor
— For mild asthma, the main lines of treatment are inhaled bronchodilators. The commonly used drugs are
  • Beta-adrenergic agonists, e.g. salbutamol, terbutaline, fenoterol
  • Anticholinergic agents, e.g. ipratropium bromide
  • Steroids, e.g. betamethasone or beclomethasone
  • Sodium cromoglycate (the latter is less effective in the older patient)
— As the elderly have problems coordinating the standard type of metered dose inhaler correctly, various devices have been invented. These include
  • 'Haleraid'

- 'The Spacer'
- 'The Volumatic'
- 'The Rota-haler'
- 'The Aerolin Auto', a breath-activated aerosol inhaler
— If inhaler therapy is technically impossible or the patient continues to have nocturnal attacks, oral bronchodilators such as theophylline or aminophylline should be considered. However, one must remember that theophylline metabolism is affected by age, smoking habits and other diseases and therefore blood concentrations should be monitored.
— Oral steroids should be used for acute asthma in short courses only. If the patient shows a good response then inhaled steroids should be substituted

CHRONIC OBSTRUCTIVE AIRWAYS DISEASE (CHRONIC AIRFLOW LIMITATION)

— This is a term that is used to apply to a range of diseases which have in common evidence of obstruction to expired airflow, e.g. chronic bronchitis and emphysema.
— Chronic bronchitis which is associated with mucous gland hypertrophy is defined by daily cough, productive of sputum, for at least 3 months in two consecutive years
— Emphysema implies dilatation of the terminal air-spaces of the lung. It can be of two types
  - Centrilobular, associated with smoking, mainly affects the centre of each lobule
  - Pan-acinar, involves the whole lobule, is severe and is associated with alpha-1-antitrypsin deficiency
— Diagnosis is usually made by exclusion. Chest X-rays are often normal, although if emphysema is present, hyperinflation, reduced lung markings and narrow vertical heart shadow may be noted. Lung function tests demonstrate obstruction with some degree of reversibility

Management
The first step of management is to prevent or limit progress of the disease by persuading the patient to stop smoking. The other measures include treatment of acute infection, bronchodilator therapy for those who have demonstrable airflow reversibility and treatment of complications such as hypoxia, cor pulmonale and polycythaemia. Hypoxia, a resting pO_2 of <55 mmHg, together with poor exercise tolerance, suggests that treatment with oxygen may be useful. These individuals should be encouraged to use oxygen at least 15 hours a day, in order to lower the incidence of cor pulmonale. If, however, despite this cor pulmonale develops it should be treated with addition of

diuretics. Polycythaemia (PCV > 60) may develop in patients with chronic airflow limitation (CAL) and lead to increased viscosity and its vascular sequelae. The incidence of these complications can be reduced by reducing the PCV by repeated venesection.

BRONCHIAL CARCINOMA

— Primary bronchial carcinoma is common in the elderly, particularly in male smokers, in those with fibrotic lung disease and those exposed to blue asbestos during their occupation.
— There are two common histological types
  • Small-cell (oat-cell) anaplastic
  • Squamous cell
— The former usually grows rapidly and metastasizes to liver, bone and brain. The latter, however, is the commoner type, grows more slowly and usually arises from a large bronchus, causing a local mass which may obstruct or cavitate

Clinical features
Typical symptoms are haemoptysis, chest pain and breathlessness. Stridor, a harsh noise audible at the mouth, usually in inspiration, or dysphagia may also occur through direct compression of the trachea or oesophagus. In addition, the elderly may present atypically with falls due to muscle weakness, peripheral neuropathy, weakness and lassitude due to hyponatraemia, hypercalcaemia or hypokalaemia, or painful wrists due to hypertrophic pulmonary osteoarthropathy or a painful arm from apical or pan-coast tumour which may cause not only arm pain with wasting of the hand muscles but ptosis as well.

Diagnosis
Diagnosis is usually made on radiology, which may include CT scanning, sputum cytology and fibre-optic bronchoscopy.

Treatment
Treatment is considered in squamous cell carcinoma if the tumour is confined and there is no invasion of extrapulmonary structures, if there are no distant metastases, and if the patient is fit and lung function tests indicate that the patient is likely to tolerate surgery. However, if these conditions are not met then chemotherapy is the treatment of choice for small-cell carcinoma and radiotherapy for non-small-cell tumour to relieve the patient's symptoms, such as bone pain, superior vena caval obstruction, compression of large airways causing stridor, dysphagia due to oesophageal compression or haemoptysis.

— Other treatments include laser therapy for stridor, local nerve block for chest wall pain and intrapleural tetracycline or talc for persistent pleural effusion, dexamethasone for

cerebral metastases, prednisolone for hypercalcaemia, tamoxifen for gynaecomastia and fluid restriction and demeclocycline for hyponatraemia.
— If the pain persists despite the above measures then the disease is too widespread for radiotherapy, and opiates should be considered with or without indomethacin or other non-steroidal anti-inflammatory agents

OTHER LUNG TUMOURS

Metastases

Blood-borne metastases can present as a single or multiple spherical shadows of any size, whereas lymphatic metastases present as linear shadowing, often with enlarged lymph nodes. Identification of the primary source is only of value if specific chemotherapy is likely to help the patient, e.g. for carcinoma of the breast, prostate or thyroid.

Lymphoma

Mediastinal or hilar nodes are commonly involved and may be complicated by pleural effusion.

Benign tumours

These are much less common than malignant tumours and include adenomas, which may present with haemoptysis or signs of bronchial obstruction. The carcinoid syndrome, which is usually associated with tumours of the terminal ileum, may occasionally be caused by a bronchial adenoma. A pulmonary hamartoma is usually an isolated solitary calcified round opacity on chest X-ray. If the patient is unfit for surgery then needle biopsy or examination of aspirated material may help to exclude malignancy or tuberculosis.

Pleural tumours

These are mostly metastatic, though if there is a history of asbestos exposure then mesothelioma should be considered. In either case the treatment is palliative.

ACUTE THROMBOEMBOLIC DISEASE

Acute thromboembolic disease is common and is often noted at autopsy in the elderly. Risk factors are surgery, particularly pelvic and hip operation, immobility, cardiac disease, malignant disease, oestrogen therapy, previous episodes of thromboembolism and cerebrovascular accidents.

Clinical presentation
The clinical presentations range between two extremes:

— Acute massive pulmonary enbolism: this may present with severe breathlessness and chest pain, or faintness on slight effort, or even a stroke. The patient is usually shocked, has right ventricular strain as well as raised jugular venous pressure

— Pulmonary infarction: smaller emboli occlude lobar or segmental blood supply to the lung. The symptoms and signs therefore resemble those of respiratory disease, such as pneumonia. The patient may complain of pleuritic chest pain, sudden breathlessness, haemoptysis and mild fever. On examination the patient has raised respiratory rate, pleural friction rub, expiratory wheeze or signs of consolidation or effusion

Investigations

— Chest X-ray may initially appear normal in massive embolism. Later on, however, when the initial clinical picture is that of pulmonary infarction, chest X-ray may show one or more areas of consolidation adjacent to the chest wall or a small effusion with elevated diaphragm. Linear shadows may also be present

— ECG, although insensitive in the elderly, may reveal signs of right ventricular strain, i.e. S1, Q3, T3, or right bundle branch block or right axis deviation

— Arterial blood gases invariably show reduction in both p_aO_2, and p_aCO_2, though similar abnormalities are also seen in pneumonia and heart failure

— Ventilation–perfusion isotope lung scan is said to be the investigation of choice; however, it has a high false-positive rate

— Pulmonary angiography should be carried out where the patient is seriously ill or if thrombolytic therapy (streptokinase or urokinase) is being considered

— Lower limb venography is sometimes valuable to ascertain whether or not there is a clot present in the deep veins, particularly if there is equivocal evidence of embolism

Management

— Patients in whom massive embolism has occurred and who are seriously ill may intially require resuscitation. Heparin therapy should be started at this stage, and if there is no rapid improvement then pulmonary angiography with a view to IV streptokinase or embolectomy must be considered in

elderly who have been 'fit' prior to acquiring the embolism.
— Anticoagulants with heparin and warfarin are conservative
  measures which prevent further venous thrombosis and
  embolism, thus allowing the normal processes of fibrinolysis
  and organization of thrombi to take place. Treatment should
  continue for at least 3 months, but longer if the patient is at
  special risk of further episodes.

BIBLIOGRAPHY

Alvarez S, Shell C, Berk S L 1987 Pulmonary tuberculosis in elderly men. American Journal
  of Medicine 82: 604–606
Chemotherapy of pulmonary tuberculosis in Britain 1988. Drugs and Therapeutics Bulletin
  261: 1–4
Fowler R 1985 Ageing and lung function. Age and Ageing 14: 209–215
Lu Y L, Chow W H, Humphries M J, Wong K W S, Gabriel M 1986 Cryptic miliary
  tuberculosis. Quarterly Journal of Medicine (New Series) 59: 421–428
Mahler D A (ed) 1986 Respiratory diseases. Clinics in Geriatric Medicine 2(2)
Petheram I S, Jones D A, Collins J V 1982 Assessment and management of acute asthma in
  the elderly: A comparison with younger asthmatics. Postgraduate Medical Journal
  58: 149–151

12. DISEASES OF GASTROINTESTINAL TRACT, LIVER AND PANCREAS

— Ageing is associated with many anatomical and physiological changes. These include:
  - Varicosities of mucosal vessels in the mouth
  - Impairment of taste
  - Reduced secretion of saliva
  - Weakness of pharyngeal muscles
  - Impaired oesophageal motility
  - Atrophic changes in stomach associated with achlorhydria
  - Reduced absorption in the small intestine
  - Increase in transit time, leading to constipation and development of diverticulae, particularly in the large intestine
— Although these changes do not produce symptoms, they can make assessment of the GI-tract disorders difficult
— With ageing, changes in the liver include reduction in liver mass, reduction in blood flow and reduction in enzyme activities. A major impact of these changes in the elderly is on drug metabolism, since the liver is one of the main organs for drug detoxification and excretion
— Three of the commonly encountered symptoms in the elderly are
  - Dysphagia
  - Constipation
  - Faecal incontinence

DYSPHAGIA

Dysphagia is defined as difficulty in swallowing or painful swallowing. It is a relatively common symptom that should always be taken seriously and warrants full assessment in the elderly, including examination of the mouth and pharynx. The causes of dysphagia are many and include not only conditions affecting the pharynx and oesophagus but also disorders of other organs (see Table 12.1).

Table 12.1 Causes of dysphagia

Oropharynx		
Local	Carcinoma	
	Pharyngeal abscess	
	Pharyngeal pouch	
	Abscess	
	Enlarged thyroid gland	
	Lymphadenopathy	
Muscle disease	Primary myositis	
	Amyloidosis	
	Thyroid disease	
	Myasthenia gravis	
Neurological	Cerebrovascular disease	
	Pseudobulbar palsy	
	Parkinson's disease	
	Motor neuron disease	
	Syringobulbia	
Oesophagus		
Local	Carcinoma	
	Peptic stricture	
	Diverticula	
	Candidiasis	
	Pill injury (potassium, tetracycline, quinidine)	
	Gastric volvulus	
Motility disorders	Achalasia	
	Diffuse spasms	
	Scleroderma	
	Abnormal upper oesophageal sphincter relaxation	
Extrinsic lesions	Lymphadenopathy	
	Dysphagia aortica	

Management

Depends on the cause of symptoms.

Investigations
— Barium swallow and meal
— Endoscopy
— Manometric studies
— Cineradiography

CONSTIPATION

Defined as straining of stool for more than 25% of the time and/or two or fewer stools per week with straining occurring either because the stools are hard and difficult to expel or because there is abnormality of anal/rectal function. The incidence of this symptom increases with age and this is supported by the increased use of laxatives by the elderly as a group.

Factors which can produce constipation are numerous and include not only lesions in the gastrointestinal tract but systemic diseases as well as drug therapy. Causes of constipation include

— Immobility
— Decreased roughage in diet
— Idiopathic megacolon
— Colonic carcinoma
— Sigmoid volvulus
— Fissure
— Colonic diverticula
— Hypothyroidism
— Hypercalcaemia
— Hypokalaemia
— Depression
— Neurological disorders
— Drugs
   • Analgesics
   • Iron preparations
   • Antidepressants
   • Phenothiazines
   • Opiates

Assessment of a patient with constipation should include dietary history, full examination including that of rectum, and investigation such as barium studies, EMG or manometric studies.

Management

Depends on the aetiology, but should also involve maximum use of normal physiology, including education about the gastrocolic reflex, benefits of regular exercise and of increased fibre in the diet. If these measures fail and the patient has idiopathic constipation, then laxatives should be given, preferably bulk-forming, on an intermittent basis.

FAECAL INCONTINENCE

One of the most important symptoms that is said to occur in about 3% of elderly living at home and up to 23–45% of elderly in long-stay geriatric wards. Causes of incontinence (see below) include not only severe impaction but also diseases of the colon or rectum as well as neurological disorders.

As in cases of constipation, the patient with faecal incontinence must be thoroughly assessed and investigated to find an underlying cause.

Treatment is aimed at correcting the major contributory factor. In those with neurogenic incontinence the symptoms can be controlled with intermittent use of laxatives and suppositories, with or without enemas, and antidiarrhoeal agents. Those 'young' elderly patients who have sphincter dysfunction may benefit from surgical reconstruction of the sphincter.

Causes of faecal incontinence are
— Impaction with overflow
— Diarrhoea from any cause
— Carcinoma of rectum
— Villous adenoma
— Rectal prolapse
— Previous surgery on rectum/anus
— Sphincter incompetence
— Pelvic floor neuropathy
— Dementia

DISORDERS OF THE OESOPHAGUS

Hiatus hernia and gastro-oesophageal reflux

The prevalence of hiatus hernia increases with age, reaching between 60–90% by the age of 70. Although it can be asymptomatic it can lead to symptoms of reflux, dysphagia, haemorrhage due to peptic ulceration of oesophagus, and volvulus of stomach in those patients in whom the whole of the stomach herniates into the thorax. Gastro-oesophageal reflux, which can occur without hiatus hernia, classically produces burning xiphisternal or retrosternal discomfort, particularly after meals, during exercise or postural change and occasionally it may produce chest pain similar to myocardial infarction. Symptoms usually improve spontaneously, although in some patients the reflux may lead to ulceration.

Diagnosis
Can be confirmed on barium swallow and oesophagoscopy.

Treatment
Simple measures like sleeping with the head of the bed raised, avoidance of stooping, reducing size of meal, weight reduction in obese patients and stopping smoking will produce beneficial effects.

Some may require a mixture of antacids taken after a meal, or a course of cimetidine 800 mg a day for a period of 4–8 weeks, or metoclopamide. Some patients, however, may require continuous therapy with H2 blocking agents for relief of gastro-oesophageal reflux.

Achalasia

A disease of unknown aetiology characterized by aperistalsis of oesophagus and defective relaxation of oesophageal sphincter. It is due to degeneration of the postganglion nerve fibres supplying the oesophageal smooth muscle. Symptoms produced by achalasia include dysphagia for liquids as well as for solids, regurgitation, weight loss and recurrent chest infections due to aspiration.

Diagnosis

Confirmed by cineradiography or by manometric studies demonstrating increased sensitivity to a cholinergic agent.

Treatment

Dilatation and cardiomyectomy. Those who are unfit for surgery should be given isosorbide dinitrate sublingually before meals.

Oesophageal spasm

Characterized by intermittent chest pain and/or dysphagia associated with abnormal peristaltic contractions on manometry or radiological examination. The chest pain may resemble myocardial infarction. Unfortunately, the manometric abnormalities noted are variable in patients and include not only interrupted peristalsis but abnormally slow distal propagation and a positive metacholine test.

Patients with mild symptoms require no treatment, but those with severe symptoms can be given isosorbide or nifedipine.

Oesophageal carcinoma

Occurs most frequently between the ages of 50 and 70 years and affects men more than women. It accounts for 1% of all cases of carcinoma. Histologically the majority of the tumours are squamous and only 10% are adenocarcinomas.

Clinical features

The main symptom is dysphagia, first for solids and later for liquids. One has to remember that dysphagia for solids is not always due to carcinoma, but may also be produced by other benign conditions, such as oesophagitis or Schatzki's ring, a thin annular structure located at the inferior margin of the oesophagus. Some patients may also develop pain in the upper epigastrium or back, regurgitation of retained food or saliva, aspiration pneumonia, weight loss and symptoms due to metastases.

Investigations

Barium swallow and oesophagoscopy with biopsy.

Treatment

Largely palliative as the tumour is diagnosed late. In early cases surgical excision is possible. Palliative measures include full-dose radiation or introduction of a tube prosthesis. The prognosis is poor, with 5-year survival rate of 7–28% depending on the site of tumour.

Oesophageal candidiasis

Most likely to occur in patients with malignant disease, in those who are immunosuppressed and in those with endocrine disorders like hypothyroidism, adrenal insufficiency and diabetes mellitus and in those with malnutrition. The symptoms, which occur in about 50% of patients with oesophageal candidiasis, include dysphagia, especially for solids, and retrosternal pain. In about 50% of patients oral candidiasis is present.

Treatment
Nystatin suspension

DISORDERS OF THE STOMACH

Erosions, which are superficial ulcers, differ from peptic ulcers as they do not penetrate the muscularis mucosa; they extend into the submucosa and are often found in association with gastritis and duodenitis.

Peptic ulcer

Peptic ulceration occurring in the oesophagus, stomach and duodenum is common. Approximately one-third of patients with duodenal ulcers are over the age of 60 years. Although some elderly have symptoms similar to the younger patients, others present atypically with non-specific symptoms like weight loss, and vomiting with vague abdominal discomfort. The complication rate in the elderly is high and at present half the perforations occur in those over 70 years of age, and in some of these patients the perforation is silent.

Investigations
Endoscopy and barium meal.

Treatment
Cimetidine 800 mg nocte or ranitidine 300 mg nocte for at least 6 weeks is recommended. The side effects of cimetidine which may occur in the elderly include mental confusion and depression. Surgery is recommended for complications or in those in whom medical treatment has failed, or if a patient with ulcer is also dependent on non-steroidal anti-inflammatory agents. The prognosis in uncomplicated peptic ulcer, including giant gastric ulcer, is good, whereas in those with complications the mortality is high.

Complication of partial gastrectomy
Partial gastrectomy as a treatment for uncomplicated peptic ulcer has become irrelevant. However, complications of gastrectomy, particularly polyagastrectomy carried out many years ago, are now frequently seen in the elderly. These include osteomalacia due to vitamin D deficiency, iron deficiency anaemia, megaloblastic anaemia and weight loss.

Gastric carcinoma

The third commonest cancer causing death in the elderly. It is most commonly seen in the sixth or seventh decade and the male : female ratio is 2 : 1. The predisposing factors include achlorhydria, pernicious anaemia and benign adenoma.

Symptoms
May resemble those of peptic ulcer, but a significant number of patients present with anorexia, progressive weight loss, epigastric discomfort or epigastric mass.

Investigations
Barium meal and endoscopy.

Treatment
Surgical by choice, but unfortunately many elderly present at a late stage and in these patients palliative treatment is all that one can offer.

Gastritis

— Incidence of gastritis increases with advancing age. Atrophic gastritis is the most common cause of hypo- or achlorhydria and is characterized by partial loss of fundic glands and a corresponding decrease in parietal cell function. The role of *Campylobacter pylori* in the pathogenesis of chronic gastritis is not clear
— Gastritis is asymptomatic and is usually thought to be due to ageing per se. However, more marked changes are seen in pathological conditions such as pernicious anaemia, iron deficiency anaemia, chronic alcoholism, viral hepatitis, after irradiation of abdomen and following gastric surgery. These patients are usually asymptomatic too, but those with pernicious anaemia and gastritis are at risk of developing malignancy and should be endoscoped regularly
— Acute gastritis may be secondary to alcohol, drugs, and especially non-steroidal anti-inflammatory agents and staphylococcal toxins
— The ratio of $PG_1 : PG_2$ (pepsinogen) is found to relate to the histological state of the gastric mucosa. Levels decrease with increasing severity of atrophic gastritis. Serum B_{12}, circulating intrinsic factor antibodies and anaemia may be observed in severe atrophic gastritis

DISORDERS OF THE SMALL INTESTINE

Malabsorption

Many conditions can lead to malabsorption in the elderly. Symptoms like diarrhoea and steatorrhoea, which are common in younger patients, are not the usual presenting features in the elderly. It is more common to find general weakness, muscle pains, general deterioration in health, weight loss or confusion as the presenting complaints. Causes of malabsorption

— Coeliac disease
— Small bowel diverticular disease (bacterial overgrowth)
— Post-gastrectomy syndrome
— Systemic sclerosis
— Amyloidosis
— Lymphoma
— Primary biliary cirrhosis
— Skin diseases

Investigations
1. Those which elucidate the cause of malabsorption, i.e. xylose absorption test, small bowel biopsy, culture of jejunal aspirate obtained at time of jejunal biopsy. ^{14}C glycocholic breath test, measurement of Sehcat (a taurine conjugate of a synthetic bile salt containing the isotope selenium -75) retention, ^{14}C triolein test as an alternative to faecal fat estimation, ERCP (endoscopic retrograde cholangiopancreatography) and ultrasound of pancreas
2. Those which elucidate nutritional deficiencies

Treatment
This consists of correcting nutrient deficiencies and specific treatment for the underlying cause, e.g. antibiotic treatment for those patients who have bacterial overgrowth in the gut, and gluten-free diet for those with coeliac disease producing severe diarrhoea and abdominal pain.

Mesenteric ischaemia

— Acute mesenteric ischaemia can result from superior mesenteric thrombosis, superior mesenteric artery embolism associated with myocardial infarction or atrial fibrillation, venous thrombosis or low cardiac output states. The main presenting symptom is abdominal pain, which is sudden in onset and localized to the epigastrium or central abdomen
— Characteristically there is discrepancy between the severity of the pain and the paucity of abdominal signs. Other presenting clinical features include nausea and vomiting, diarrhoea (which may be bloody, although this is rare), increasing abdominal distension, absent bowel sounds and circulatory collapse, particularly at later stages
— In chronic intestinal ischaemia the patients present with recurrent acute abdominal pain which occurs 10–15 minutes after eating. The pain gradually increases in severity, reaches a plateau and then slowly disappears in 1–3 hours. The pain is mostly cramping in nature and is localized to the upper abdomen. As the pain is related to meals it leads to fear of eating, i.e. 'small meal syndrome'

Diagnosis

In both conditions diagnosis is made on clinical features but can be confirmed by arteriography in patients with suspected chronic ischaemia or in patients with acute ischaemia due to embolism. Unfortunately, in some, the diagnosis is only made at laparotomy or at autopsy.

Treatment

— Acute ischaemia: embolectomy or arterial reconstruction and excision of necrotic bowel
— Chronic ischaemia: by-pass surgery to improve blood flow. The prognosis in these patients is good.

Crohn's disease

Like ulcerative colitis, Crohn's disease has a bimodal distribution, with a second peak of incidence occurring at the age of 70 years.

Clinical features

These include gastrointestinal symptoms like diarrhoea, abdominal pain, anal symptoms or unexplained systemic symptoms like confusion. Diagnosis may be difficult because of higher prevalence of diverticular disease. The part of the bowel that is commonly involved is the ileum, with or without spread to the right side of the colon. In about 40% the distal colon is involved. The course of disease depends on the site of the bowel involved. Those patients with ileal disease tend to develop complications or features such as obstruction or peritonitis that require laparotomy, whereas those with distal colonic disease rarely come to surgery.

Treatment

— Acute attacks require treatment similar to ulcerative colitis, i.e. sulphasalazine with or without corticosteroids. Those with colonic or perianal disease may also benefit from metronidazole. Azathioprine has also been found to be useful in improving fistulae and having some value as a steroid-sparing drug. Controversy still persists as far as maintenance therapy or therapy during remission is concerned. Surgery is required for those patients who develop complications like peritonitis, fistulae or abscess. Colostomy is sometimes used to 'rest' the bowel in patients who do not respond as quickly as expected to medical treatment
— In addition to specific treatment, metabolic problems such as malnutrition, anaemia, fluid and electrolyte abnormalities should be corrected

DISORDERS OF THE LARGE INTESTINE

Pseudomembranous colitis

— Antibiotic-associated colitis or pseudomembranous colitis is due to proliferation of *Clostridium difficile* in the colon. It occurs when the normal flora has been suppressed by a broad-spectrum antibiotic
— The patient usually presents with diarrhoea without bleeding or fever. Associated with this there may be low albumin and leucocytosis. Diagnosis can be made by culturing the *Clostridium difficile* from the faeces, by detecting the toxin or by the appearance of patchy exudative membranes which are easily scraped from the red but non-friable mucosa on sigmoidoscopy.

Treatment
Consists of stopping the offending antibiotic, rehydration and use of vancomycin 125 mg qds or metronidazole.

Ulcerative colitis

A condition which has a bimodal incidence, with second peak occurring after the age of 50. The disease varies in its extent and severity. The disease in the majority is confined to the rectum but it can spread slowly to involve the rest of the colon. The risk of developing malignancy is low in the first 10 years but this risk is higher in those with extensive disease. The complications that are dangerous in the elderly are toxic dilatation and perforation. The clinical features in the elderly may be no different from younger patients and the diagnosis is confirmed by barium enema, sigmoidoscopy and biopsy.

Treatment
As in younger patients, this consists of using sulphasalazine and steroids locally or orally for acute exacerbations and sulphasalazine for prevention of relapse. Surgical treatment is indicated if the medical treatment fails or the patient has had extensive disease for 10 years and therefore has increased risk of developing malignancy, or if the patient develops acute dilatation of the colon.

Ischaemic colitis

Ischaemia of the colon is the commonest vascular disorder of the intestine in the elderly. Splenic flexure and left colon are the most commonly involved areas. The ischaemia can be due to occlusion of the large artery, venous occlusion and vascular insufficiency caused by increased intraluminal pressure and low cardiac output state. Occasionally it may be associated with other obstructive lesions, e.g. carcinoma of the colon, volvulus, faecal impaction and diverticulitis.

Clinical features

Manifestations vary

1. Gangrene of the colon presenting with abdominal pain and diarrhoea, with or without rectal bleeding
2. Acute non-gangrenous transient ischaemic colitis. The patient presents with a short history of left-sided or lower abdominal pain followed by diarrhoea mixed with bright red or dark blood. Associated features include nausea, vomiting, fever, tachycardia, left-sided tenderness and guarding
3. Non-resolving ischaemic colitis — this produces persistent diarrhoea with occasional blood loss. Ischaemic strictures, usually in the splenic flexure, can occur

Diagnosis

Diagnosis can be made on

— Barium enema in non-gangrenous colonic ischaemia: it reveals thumb-printing or macropseudopolyps
— By sigmoidoscopy and colonoscopy

Treatment

— Laparotomy for excision of dead bowel or in those with stricture
— In patients with colonic ischaemia without peritonitis: replacement of fluids, antibiotic treatment to prevent sepsis and decompression of colon if it becomes dilated. Symptoms due to reversible causes of ischaemia usually improve within days. If, however, symptoms do not improve or the condition of the patient starts to deteriorate, surgery should be carried out

Sigmoid volvulus

This often occurs in patients with chronic hepatitis and mental illness. The patient presents with abdominal distension, which can be minimal, abdominal pain and constipation. The mortality is high because of delay in recognition of the condition. In the majority of cases this can be decompressed by sigmoidoscopy or colonoscopy. If bowel strangulation occurs, surgery is mandatory.

Diverticular disease

This is a common condition which causes major disability in the elderly. The prevalence rises from 18% in the age-group 40–59 years to 42% in those over the age of 80 years.

Clinical features

— Lower abdominal pain in 78%
— Constipation, diarrhoea in 9%
— Rectal bleeding in 3%
— A palpable mass in left iliac fossa

— nausea and vomiting in 2%
— Faecal incontinence and urinary symptoms

Complications
— Perforation with peritonitis
— Abscess formation
— Fistula into bladder or vagina
— Obstruction

Treatment
Uncomplicated cases should be treated by increasing the fibre intake by 5–20 g/day. Diverticulitis should be treated with antibiotics but other complications require surgery.

Carcinoma of colon and rectum

This is a common malignancy of the elderly, the incidence of which increases with age. The predisposing conditions include ulcerative colitis, polyp or adenoma. Presenting clinical features may include diarrhoea, faecal incontinence, abdominal pain, abdominal mass or rectal bleeding, or iron deficiency anaemia. Investigations for the suspected colonic carcinoma include barium enema, sigmoidoscopy or colonoscopy.

Treatment
Surgery. The 5-year survival varies from 64 to 80%.

Angiodysplasia of colon

This is a vascular malformation which often presents with iron deficiency anaemia. The diagnosis is made by direct colonoscopy or by mesenteric arteriography.

Treatment
Diathermy via a colonoscope or surgical excision.

Intestinal pseudo-obstruction

This condition results from abnormality of intestinal motility and leads to clinical features of obstruction. The patient may be in hospital or at home with some other illness and not infrequently he or she may be dehydrated or mildly uraemic. The disorders which may produce intestinal pseudo-obstruction include
— Diabetes mellitus
— Amyloid
— Drugs with atropine-like action
— Myxoedema
— Hypoparathyroidism
— Scleroderma
— Previous abdominal irradiation
— Heavy metal poisoning

— Polymyositis
— Varicella

Treatment

— Finding the treatable cause and removing it
— Reducing gaseous distension
— Correcting fluid and electrolyte abnormalities
— Combating bacterial overgrowth as abnormal growth may contribute to reduced and abnormal motility
— Stimulating intestinal motility by using drugs like prostigmine

If the colon is grossly distended then decompression by colonoscope may be required.

DISORDERS OF THE LIVER

Chronic active hepatitis

— Characterized by piecemeal necrosis with associated bridging necrosis or multilobular collapse with lymphocytic and plasma cell infiltration
— Associated with these changes two-thirds of the patients have smooth muscle antibodies in the blood. Although this is predominantly a disease of younger people there is another peak after the menopause. Histological changes of chronic active hepatitis may be found in association with ulcerative colitis or following exposure to certain drugs, e.g. methyldopa, isoniazid, nitrofurantoin, oxyphenistan, ketoconazole

Treatment

As the course of disease is variable treatment with steroids should only be used in those who have symptoms. Patients should be monitored regularly with clinical evaluation, biochemical measures and if necessary by biopsy. Patients with severe disease may require long-term steroid therapy.

Primary biliary cirrhosis

Although typically this occurs in middle-aged females it is also found in the elderly. Clinical features which the patient may have include pruritus, skin pigmentation, jaundice, malabsorption syndrome, finger clubbing, xanthoma, enlarged liver with smooth edge, splenomegaly, presence of mitochondrial antibodies and raised IgM levels or raised serum alkaline phosphatase. Some patients may also have features suggesting the involvement of other systems, e.g. CRST syndrome (calcinosis, Raynaud's disease, sclerodactyly, telangiectasia), thyroid disease or Sjogren's syndrome.

Treatment

The elderly are often asymptomatic and therefore require no treatment. Those with jaundice should be given fat-soluble vitamins A, D (to prevent osteomalacia) and K, calcium supplements and cholestyramine to relieve pruritus.

Cirrhosis

In the elderly this presents with a clinical picture similar to that which occurs in younger patients. It may follow viral hepatitis, alcoholism, disturbed immunity, prolonged cholestasis, iron overload, malnutrition, jejuno-ileal by-pass, or it may occur as cryptogenic cirrhosis in which the aetiology is not clear.

DISORDERS OF THE GALL BLADDER AND BILIARY TRACT

Gallstones

The incidence of cholelithiasis increases with age and the condition is found at autopsy in about one-third of elderly over the age of 70 years. However, only a small number during life have symptoms, which may include mild jaundice of short duration, severe obstructive jaundice, cholecystitis, cholangitis or biliary colic. Investigations of choice are ultrasound and ERCP. In some patients cholangiography may be required.

Treatment

This depends on localization of stones, type of stones, biliary tract complications and general health of the patient. For radiolucent gallstones in a functioning gall bladder ursodeoxycholic acid or chenodeoxycholic acid should be tried for dissolution of stones. In those patients with radiopaque stones who have had an attack of cholecystitis or cholangitis, cholecystectomy should be carried out. For the frail patient who is not fit for general anaesthesia but who has obstructive jaundice, ERCP with papillotomy is the treatment of choice.

Carcinoma of the gall bladder

This is a disease of elderly females, with a frequency of 0.2–5%. There is a close association with gallstones. It usually presents with obstructive jaundice, right upper quadrant pain and weight loss. On examination there is usually a hard mass palpable in the right hypochondrium. Investigations of choice are ultrasound and ERCP.

Treatment

Surgical, but unfortunately prognosis is poor, with 85% dying within a year of presentation. In some patients only palliative measures like insertion of prosthesis to relieve jaundice is possible, as the tumour is found to be unresectable.

Carcinoma of the bile duct

This condition tends to affect males more than females. The presenting clinical features include obstructive jaundice, which is occasionally intermittent, pain, weight loss and marked hepatomegaly. Diagnosis is usually made by ERCP. Prognosis depends on the site of the tumour. Patients with tumours arising from the ampulla fare better than with those arising from the rest of the biliary tract, in whom the maximum benefit is only obtained from palliative measures and/or radiotherapy.

DISORDERS OF THE PANCREAS

Acute pancreatitis

The occurrence of pancreatitis is two to three times higher in those above the age of 50 years than in younger people. The clinical features include epigastric pain with radiation into the back, vomiting, confusion or unconsciousness, occasional pleural effusion or even an abnormal electrocardiograph. Investigations may reveal raised serum amylase (if this is measured later in the course of the disease it can be normal), raised lipase, raised blood sugar and raised bilirubin. Aetiological factors include gallstones, ischaemia, hypothermia and carbon monoxide poisoning. It is associated with a high mortality in the elderly.

Treatment
Replacement of fluids, analgesia and aspiration of duodenum. Lapafotomy should be carried out in those patients who develop complications like pancreatic abscess or pseudocyst.

Chronic pancreatitis

Usually the end result of repeated episodes of acute pancreatitis. The clinical features include pain, nausea and vomiting in half the patients, weight loss, diarrhoea (although this is less frequent than it is in younger patients) and glycosuria (which tends to occur twice as frequently in the old as in the young). Investigations which lead to the confirmation of the diagnosis include plain abdominal X-rays, which may show calcification, and the Lundh test, which demonstrates reduced tryptic activity.

Treatment
Pancreatic extract in those with severe diarrhoea or malabsorption.

Pancreatic carcinoma

This has peak incidence in the elderly over 80 years, and the classical presentation is with painless obstructive jaundice. The other features that patients may have include anorexia, weight loss, liver enlargement, melaena and deep vein thrombosis. Investigations of choice are ultrasound and ERCP.

Treatment
Usually pancreatic carcinoma presents late and only palliative treatment to relieve jaundice can be carried out. The prognosis is poor.

BIBLIOGRAPHY

Castell D O 1988 Dysphagia in the elderly. Journal of the American Geriatrics Society 34: 248–249

Drugs and Therapeutics Bulletin 1986 Peptic ulcer: Which patients to consider for surgery, 24: 77–78

Dudley H A F, Paterson-Brown S 1986 Pseudo-obstruction. British Medical Journal 292: 1157–1158

Hellemans J, Vantrappen G (eds) 1984 Gastrointestinal tract disorders in the elderly. Churchill Livingstone, Edinburgh

Krasinki S D, Russel R M, Samloff M et al 1986 Fundic atrophic gastritis in elderly population. Effect on haemoglobin and several nutritional indicators. Journal of the American Geriatrics Society 34: 800–806

Rhodes J, Rose J 1985 Crohn's disease in the elderly. British Medical Journal 291: 1149–1150

Vallon A G, Crocker J R 1985 Obstructive jaundice in the elderly. Age and Ageing 14: 143–148

13. RENAL DISEASE

— Renal function and structure deteriorate with increasing age. The renal mass falls from 250–270 g in young adulthood to 180–200 g by the age of 90. Glomeruli fall by 30–50% and there is associated increase in sclerotic glomeruli. As a result of this, there is a fall in glomerular filtration rate, which declines from its maximum at the age of 30 (140 ml/min per 1.75 m^2) by 1% per year

— These changes do not alter serum creatinine or urea, but do make renal function more vulnerable to stress

URINARY TRACT INFECTION

Bactiuria

Twenty per cent of healthy women and 10% of men over the age of 65 years have bactiuria. The significance of this in women is uncertain but in those with indwelling catheters and in those women with underlying malignancy it is said to be associated with increased mortality.

Symptomatic lower urinary tract infection

As in younger patients, this may present with dysuria, frequency and haematuria, or it may present with incontinence or confusion.

Diagnosis
Confirmed by microscopy and culture.

Treatment
With appropriate antibiotic for 5–7 days.

Pyelonephritis

This is more serious and implies infection of the renal parenchyma and pelvis. It may result in septicaemia or renal failure.

Predisposing conditions include

— Lower urinary tract infection

— Lower urinary tract obstruction
— Renal stone disease
— Neurological disease which interferes with bladder emptying
— Anatomical abnormalities of the renal tract

One method of differentiating pyelonephritis from lower urinary tract infection is to detect antibody-coated bacteria in the urine. The patient may present with malaise, dehydration, fever, loin pain and tenderness, frequency, dysuria or confusion.

Treatment

Bed rest, fluids and antibiotics as well as investigations to exclude an underlying cause.

CHRONIC RENAL FAILURE

This is a common problem in the elderly which is associated with disappointing outcome. The clinical picture is pleomorphic and the severity of symptoms varies according to the degree of uraemia.

The features (involving different systems) which may be present include
— Cardiovascular
  • Hypertension
  • Congestive cardiac failure
  • Pericarditis
  • Retinopathy including macular star
— Gastrointestinal
  • Nausea
  • Vomiting
  • Hiccups
  • Blood loss due to colitis
— Respiratory
  • Kussmaul's respiration
  • Respiratory tract infection
— Blood
  • Anaemia
  • Leucopenia
  • Thrombocytopaenia
  • Qualitative defect in platelet function
— Neuromuscular
  • Peripheral neuropathy
  • Myopathy
  • Muscular twitching
  • Convulsions
  • Confusion

— Skin
  • Dry with yellowish/brownish pigmentation
  • Occasionally pruritus due to 'urea frost'

Causes

— Obstructive uropathy: commonest cause
— Interstitial nephritis/chronic pyelonephritis
— Nephrosclerosis
— Amyloid
— Diabetic nephropathy
— Hypertension
— Multiple myeloma
— Collagen vascular disease
— Polycystic renal disease: adult type with dominant inheritance

Management

— To establish a definitive diagnosis by history, physicial examination and investigations directed to the causes outlined above
— Treatment of infection if present
— Assessment and treatment of fluid deficit
— Treatment of electrolyte abnormalities
— Treatment of hypertension if present
— Treatment of retention of uric acid by allopurinol
— Protein restriction to 0.5 g/kg body weight to prolong the life of endogenous kidney
— Treatment of osteodystrophy with vitamin D analogues and consideration of dialysis, i.e. haemodialysis or continuous ambulatory peritoneal dialysis. CAPD is probably best suited for the elderly

ACUTE RENAL FAILURE

The elderly are more susceptible to acute renal failure than younger persons, as the aged kidneys are much less able to respond to changes in blood pressure, water load or solute load. Acute renal failure is defined as a sudden fall in glomerular filtration, usually accompanied by oliguria, i.e. urine output of 400 ml per 24 hours. The causes can be divided into three main groups:

1. Pre-renal: resulting from hypotension from any cause, e.g. cardiogenic shock, septic shock and intravascular contraction, as in blood loss and saline depletion. The commonest cause in the elderly is dehydration due to infection, diuretics or diabetes mellitus

2. Renal: this may follow from the above (acute tubular nephropathy) or result from renal artery and venous occlusion, acute glomerulonephritis, acute interstitial nephropathy, nephrotoxins including drugs, exacerbation of chronic renal failure, etc.
3. Post-renal: the commonest cause of obstructed uropathy in men is prostatic hypertrophy, and in women procidentia. In the case of the latter 40% of females with third-degree prolapse have an obstructed uropathy, in which the presence of infection can lead to acute renal failure. Acute renal failure may also result from ureteric obstruction secondary to calculi, sloughed papillae or even a tumour

Management

The first step is to establish a diagnosis and to categorize the patient into the groups outlined above, since the treatment varies according to the cause. Most cases, however, will be pre-renal and can be diagnosed by examining the urine to plasma ratio for urea and osmolarity. In general, pre-renal values for urine to plasma ratio of urea and creatinine is >7:1, whereas in established renal failure it is <7:1. Urine osmolality in pre-renal failure is usually >600 mosmol/kg, whereas it is 300–400 mosmol/kg in established renal failure. Obstructive uropathy is best diagnosed by ultrasound of the abdomen, and if the renal tract is dilated then the treatment is to confirm the site of obstruction and surgery, provided there is still renal function present. Small kidneys on ultrasound usually equate with acute or chronic renal failure.

— In pre-renal causes, expansion of intravascular volume by appropriate fluid, e.g. blood in cases of severe haemorrhage, or saline in cases of severe sodium loss
— In renal causes it is important to correct the volume depletion if present, treat the precipitating cause and remove any underlying potentially toxic agents. It is worth giving a challenge of fluids and diuretics until it is clear that the acute renal failure is established. In the latter case there is no point in giving increasing amounts of diuretics in the hope of producing diuresis
— Treatment should be carried out in a high-dependency environment and should include restriction of protein, potassium and fluid (intake equal to renal output + insensible loss). If the patient's condition starts to deteriorate, i.e. he or she develops encephalopathy, increasing potassium, acidosis, fluid overload or rising urea, the patient should be dialysed
— Renal biopsy should be considered in patients with unexplained renal failure, as it has been shown that treatable conditions may be picked up

RENAL CARCINOMA

This is a disease of the middle-aged and elderly, and the highest incidence is in the 50–70-year age group. It may present with haematuria (present in 35% of cases), mass in the loin, pyrexia of unknown origin, solitary pulmonary mass, polycythaemia, pathological fractures or non-specific symptoms of malignancy such as weight loss, malaise, ill health, anaemia or raised ESR.

Management
Management is to make a diagnosis on history, physical examination and investigations, which include ultrasound or CT scan. In addition bone scan may be needed to detect secondary spread. Once a definitive diagnosis has been made, nephrectomy should be considered in all patients as metastases have a tendency to disappear after the primary tumour has been removed, particularly if these are localized to the soft tissue. A solitary metastatic lesion should be resected or treated with radiation. Radiotherapy and chemotherapy can be used to treat residual disease if present.

NEPHROTIC SYNDROME

This is an entity that is not often considered in the differential diagnosis of oedema in the elderly. Although uncommon, it does occur. It is a clinical syndrome which has features of proteinuria of <3.5 g per 24 hours per 1.73 m^2 body surface area, hypoalbuminaemia and hypercholesterolaemia, with fluid and salt retention.

Causes
— Membranous glomerulonephritis
— Minimal-change glomerulonephritis
— Diabetic nephropathy
— Collagen vascular disease, e.g. RA, SLE
— Proliferative glomerulonephritis
— Interstitial nephritis
— Amyloid: accounts for 20% of total causes of nephrotic syndrome in those over 50 years of age
— Thrombosis of renal vein
— Drugs, e.g. penicillamine, gold
— Heavy metal poisoning, e.g. mercury, lead
— Chronic infection, e.g. malaria, syphilis

Although membranous glomerulonephritis is the commonest cause in the elderly, minimal change can also occur, particularly in those with diabetes mellitus. It is because of this that it is important that renal biopsy is carried out to make an accurate diagnosis, since minimal-change glomerulonephritis may respond to steroids.

Management

The main essentials are
1. High-protein and high-calorie diet with salt restriction
2. Bed rest when fluid retention is gross
3. Diuretics, usually in combination of loop diuretic and spironolactone
4. Treatment of complications such as infection or venous thrombosis
5. Corticosteroids and immunosuppressive drugs in those with treatable causes

PROSTATIC HYPERTROPHY

Frequency of prostatic hypertrophy increases from 30% in the seventh decade to 100% in the tenth. Although pathogenesis is unclear it is unknown to occur in patients who have been castrated before the age of 40 years. It is the commonest cause of difficulty in micturition in men and the symptoms may include urinary frequency, nocturia, urgency and/or incontinence, difficulty in passing urine, dribbling, urine infection, acute retention or chronic retention with or without overflow and renal failure. Sometimes, however, patients may have very few symptoms and the only indication of retention with overflow may be nocturnal enuresis.

Management

Surgical relief of the obstruction by transurethral resection or open prostatectomy and treatment of any underlying complications.

PROSTATIC CARCINOMA

This is a very common hormone-dependent malignancy of men, with a prevalence increasing rapidly after the age of 70 years. Patients may present with symptoms of prostatism, bone pain due to secondaries, retention of urine, signs of spinal cord or root compression or renal failure, or with non-specific symptoms such as weight loss, anaemia or lethargy. Occasionally they may also present with symptoms of osteomalacia which results from hypophosphataemia due to renal tubular loss of phosphate. In this situation, the patient has low plasma phosphate with a low renal phosphate threshold concentration. Some of the symptoms in these patients respond well to vitamin D.

Management

Transrectal prostatic biopsy to confirm diagnosis, assess renal tract for evidence of obstruction, measure acid and alkaline phosphatase, bone scan to assess the extent of bony metastases and resection of the prostate gland.

Hormonal therapy is reserved mainly for those with metastatic disease. The main aim of hormonal therapy is to reduce testosterone production, either by orchidectomy or by exogenous oestrogens, or with the use of gonadotrophin releasing hormone analogues. The initial treatment should be with low doses of stilboestrol (1 mg/day) or cyproterone acetate, as the latter has fewer side effects but the same efficacy as other modes of treatment. Recently, there has been some success with the use of the antifungal drug ketoconazole, which inhibits the synthesis of androgens. In addition to hormonal therapy, if the patient has only a single painful deposit then radiotherapy should be considered.

Prognosis

Usually related to the cell type, i.e. degree of differentiation and clinical stage. The mean survival for stage 4 is 2 years. The progress of the disease, particularly in those with bony secondaries, can be measured with the use of computerized bone scan.

BIBLIOGRAPHY

Anderson S, Brenner B M 1987 The ageing kidney: Structure, function, mechanisms and therapeutic implications. Journal of the American Geriatrics Society 35: 590–593

Drelichman A, Decker D A, Al-Sarraf M, Vaitkevicius V K, Muz J 1984 Computerised bone scan: A potentially useful technique to measure response in prostatic carcinoma. Cancer 53: 1061–1068

Frocht A, Fillit H 1984 Renal disease in the geriatric patient. Journal of the American Geriatrics Society 32: 28–43

McInnes E G, Levy D W, Chaudhuri M D, Bhah G L 1987 Renal failure in the elderly. Quarterly Journal of Medicine (new series) 64: 583–588

Murphy P J, Wright G, Rai G S 1987 Nephrotic syndrome in the elderly. Journal of the American Geriatrics Society 35: 170–173

Zech P, Colon S, Pointet P, Deteix P, Labeeum M, Leitienne P 1982. The nephrotic syndrome in adults aged over 60: Aetiology, evolution and treatment of 76 cases. Clinical Nephrology 18: 232–236

14. HAEMATOLOGICAL DISORDERS

Although there is a fall in haemoglobin with age, it is important to remember that anaemia is not a physiological phenomenon but a pathological entity. It is often a presenting sign of a serious underlying illness. The reported prevalence of anaemia in community surveys varies from 2.4 to 21% and in hospitalized elderly from 6.4 to 14% depending on the level of haemoglobin used to define anaemia.

IRON DEFICIENCY ANAEMIA

This is the most frequent type of anaemia found in the elderly and is present in 45–70% of cases of anaemia. The cause of iron deficiency in the majority of cases is blood loss, the site of blood loss being the gastrointestinal tract, genitourinary tract or, less frequently, another site. In the GI tract the lesions commonly found are oesophagitis, haemorrhagic gastritis, gastric polyp, gastric ulcer, gastric carcinoma, duodenal ulcer, gastric erosions induced by drugs such as non-steroidal anti-inflammatory agents, caecal carcinoma and colonic carcinoma. In some patients the iron deficiency anaemia may be associated with carcinoma without any evidence of blood loss, or general medical conditions like rheumatoid arthritis, malnutrition or malabsorption.

— Often the elderly present in a non-specific manner leading to self-neglect (failure to thrive), falls, apathy or increasing confusion. Dyspnoea, dizziness and tiredness — typical features of anaemia — may also occur in some patients with severe anaemia

Diagnosis
The diagnosis of iron deficiency in elderly patients is suggested by a blood film showing hypochromia, microcytosis with anisocytosis and poikilocytosis. The serum iron level is low and the total iron binding capacity high in the majority of the patients. In some both serum iron and TIBC (total iron binding capacity) can be normal. In these individuals the diagnosis can be confirmed by:

— Bone marrow examination to show absent or reduced iron stores

    — Low ferritin values
    — Positive response to treatment

Treatment

Oral therapy with ferrous sulphate is the treatment of choice, but if the patient cannot tolerate this or be relied upon to comply with oral therapy, he or she should be given iron by parenteral infusion. The latter can be organized in the day hospital, where a patient can be given a test dose prior to infusion.

MACROCYTOSIS AND MEGALOBLASTIC ANAEMIA

— Mean corpuscular volume (MCV) increases slightly but significantly with age. Macrocytosis is suggested to be the hallmark of uncomplicated folic acid or vitamin B_{12} deficiency and may precede the onset of anaemia by months or years. On the other hand, some authors have concluded that elevated values can be found without any obvious pathological causes and one of the benign factors that may cause a rise in MCV in humans is smoking

— The reported incidence of macrocytosis varies from 1.4 to 4% in patients admitted to hospital

— The causes of macrocytosis without megaloblastic change in bone marrow are many
    • Alcoholism
    • Liver disease
    • Hypothyroidism
    • Myelodysplastic syndrome
    • Haemolytic anaemia
    • IgG Monoclonal gammopathy
    • Haemorrhage
    • Waldenstrom's macroglobulinaemia
    • Leucoerythroblastic anaemia
    • Anticonvulsant therapy
    • Cytotoxic therapy
    • Sideroblastic anaemia

— In the majority of cases the cause is found to be one of the non-haematological disorders. On the other hand, nearly all patients with macrocytosis and megaloblastic change in bone marrow have either B_{12} deficiency or folic acid deficiency or deficiency of both B_{12} and folic acid. The causes of deficiency of Vitamin B_{12} and folic acid are listed in Table 14.1. Although most patients with folic acid or B_{12} deficiency or both have macrocytosis and anaemia, one has to remember that some patients with these deficiencies may not have macrocytosis. The conditions which may result in

Table 14.1 Causes of B_{12} and folic acid deficiency

B_{12} deficiency	Folic acid deficiency

Pernicious anaemia
Gastrectomy
Malabsorption
	Malnutrition
	Malabsorption
	Excessive demands, e.g.
	   Malignancy
	   Haemolytic anaemia
	   Chronic inflammatory disease

Ileal disease	Drugs
	   Anticonvulsants
	   Trimethoprim

masking of macrocytosis include coexisting iron deficiency, infection, inflammation, renal failure and thalassaemia. In these individuals the deficiency is suggested by hypersegmentation of neutrophil nuclei. Serum B_{12} and folic acid levels again can be normal in the presence of deficiency state, and in these individuals replacement with B_{12} and/or folic acid results in MCV falling to within normal range. On the other hand, low serum B_{12} value does not itself mean that the patient has pernicious anaemia

LEUCOERYTHROBLASTIC ANAEMIA

This is defined as anaemia associated with immature red and white cells in the peripheral blood film. Until recently it was thought to be almost diagnostic of bone marrow infiltration, but studies since 1963 have shown that some benign conditions are also associated with this blood picture. Some of these include infection, iron deficiency, B_{12} or folic acid deficiency, recent haemorrhage, coeliac disease and heart failure.

HAEMOLYTIC ANAEMIA

— One of the diagnostic features of haemolytic anaemia is the presence of reticulocytosis. The common type of haemolytic anaemia found in the elderly is the auto-immune haemolytic anaemia, which may be associated with cold antibodies of IgM type
— Haemolytic anaemia can be idiopathic or associated with an underlying disease such as myelofibrosis, malignant lymphoma, collagenoses, ulcerative colitis, mycoplasma pneumoniae or secondary to drugs such as methyldopa, penicillin, salicylates, phenacetin, etc. Direct Coombs' test

in idiopathic haemolytic anaemia is usually positive.
Prognosis depends on the aetiology, the type of anaemia
and the titre of antibodies
— Treatment with steroids will benefit those with warm
antibodies in the serum. Those with cold antibodies may
show little or no response

SIDEROBLASTIC ANAEMIA

— This is a diserythropoietic disorder in which there is
impaired utilization of iron. The diagnostic feature is the
presence of increased numbers of ringed sideroblasts
(nucleated red cell precursors containing iron granules
arranged in a perinuclear ring) in the bone marrow. On the
blood film the picture resembles iron deficiency anaemia but
the serum iron and TIBC are usually normal and there is no
response to treatment with iron
— It can be primary or secondary. In primary sideroblastic
anaemia the red cells may be macrocytic rather than
microcytic, serum iron may be normal or raised, TIBC is
often reduced and serum ferritin is high. Often these
patients require no treatment as the haemoglobin is
maintained. Those who develop overt clinical anaemia may
show some response to pyridoxine 100–1000 mg a day with
folic acid. Some cases after several years terminate in acute
myeloblastic or myelomonocytic leukaemia. Secondary
acquired sideroblastic anaemia may be produced by any one
of the following
  - Drugs, e.g. PAS, isoniazid, cycloserine, paracetamol,
    chloramphenicol
  - Lead poisoning
  - Myeloproliferative disorders
  - Myeloma
  - Carcinoma
  - Collagen diseases
  - Myxoedema
  - Malabsorption
  - Partial gastrectomy
  - Alcoholism

MYELODYSPLASTIC SYNDROME

— Myelodysplastic syndromes are characterized by anaemia,
refractory to haematinic replacements. Five types of

syndrome have been described and these include
- Refractory anaemia (RA)
- Refractory anaemia with ring sideroblasts
- Refractory anaemia with excess of blasts
- Chronic myelomonocytic leukaemia
- Refractory anaemia with excess of blasts in transformation

— The anaemia may be associated with neutropenia and/or thrombocytopenia. Gross enlargement of liver, spleen and lymph nodes is not found, although mild enlargement of spleen may occur in 5–30% of patients. The bone marrow is hypercellular, with morphological abnormalities being present in all cell lines, and this may lead to the presence of ring sideroblasts. The clinical course is chronic and variable and some patients require repeated blood transfusions for anaemia. Survival ranges from a few months to 15 years. Death usually results from complication of neutropenia or thrombocytopenia or from acute leukaemic crisis. The occurrence of other cancers in patients with myelodysplastic syndrome is also increased

NORMOCHROMIC NORMOCYTIC ANAEMIA

This is defined as anaemia associated with normal morphology on blood film. Serum iron, B_{12} and red cell folate are normal in these individuals. The conditions in which the normochromic normocytic anaemia may be found include
— Renal failure
— Malignancy
— Rheumatoid arthritis
— Hypothyroidism
— Bacterial endocarditis
— Liver disease
— Collagen disease
— Haemolytic anaemia
— Alcoholism
— Scurvy
— Varicose ulcers
— Pressure sores

Treatment is that of the underlying condition or disorder.

LEUKAEMIAS

Chronic lymphatic leukaemia (CLL)

This is one of the commonest lymphoproliferative disorders that occurs in the elderly. The incidence increases with age. Usually patients present insidiously with increasing fatigue, loss of appetite, lymphadenopathy, recurrent infections or attacks of herpes zoster. In some the disease may be asymptomatic and picked up on routine blood count, which reveals an increased number of lymphocytes. In the majority, lymphocytes are of B-cells and only in 1–2% is the leukaemia of T-cell origin. Although hypogammaglobulinaemia in CLL is a common occurrence, gamma-globulins may be increased. The other associations include low ESR, and autoimmune haemolytic anaemia with positive Coombs' test. The cause of the illness is variable.

Treatment

Asymptomatic cases require no treatment. Those with symptoms and hepatosplenomegaly can be given chlorambucil 2–8 mg a day with prednisolone 40 mg a day if anaemia, particularly haemolytic anaemia, is present. Radiotherapy for local deposits or painful lymph nodes has also been found to be useful.

Prolymphocytic leukaemia

This is an unusual condition occurring predominantly in elderly men. It lies between CLL and lymphosarcoma cell leukaemia. Clinical features include massive splenomegaly with little or no lymphadenopathy, and high white cell count in peripheral blood consisting of prolymphocytes.

Hairy cell leukaemia

This accounts for about 2% of all leukaemias. Patients often present with leucopenia, thrombocytopenia, anaemia and splenomegaly. A characteristic feature is the presence of mononuclear cells with pseudopodia and numerous short villi around the cytoplasm of the membrane.

Chronic myeloid leukaemia

Although common in the young, this can occur in the elderly. Some present atypically with minimal or no hepatosplenomegaly, not so high white cell count, increased platelet count and increased alkaline phosphatase instead of being reduced. Treatment is the same as in younger patients, i.e. busulphan.

POLYCYTHAEMIA

— This is a myeloproliferative disorder characterized by increased red cell mass. It may be primary (polycythaemia rubra vera) or secondary due to hypoxia in patients with chronic lung disease or acquired heart disease, or

secondary to renal carcinoma, polycystic disease or cerebellar haemangioblastoma or ovarian carcinoma
— The peak incidence of primary polycythaemia rubra vera is 50–80 years. Symptoms can be non-specific but when present they are produced by increased blood volume and viscosity, i.e. cerebral ischaemia or thrombosis, myocardial infarction or peripheral vascular disease. Other presenting features include pruritus, which occurs in two-thirds of cases, peptic ulceration, bleeding tendency and gout. Clinical signs include enlarged spleen, plethoric facies and peripheral cyanosis
— Investigations reveal raised haemoglobin, raised packed cell volume and red cell mass

Treatment
Phosphorus-32 (^{32}P) by choice, although busulphan or chlorambucil can be used in some patients.

PLATELET DISORDERS

Thrombocythaemia

This may occur in the elderly without shortening life. Clinical features include tendency to bleeding, thrombosis, splenomegaly, platelet counts of greater than one million, and abnormal platelet forms, with some showing abnormal function.

Treatment
With ^{32}P or busulphan. As an entity this may have to be distinguished from thrombocytosis, which can be found in association with other systemic conditions.

Causes of thrombocytosis
— Haemorrhage
— Splenectomy
— Chronic inflammatory disease
— Malignancy
— Chronic renal failure
— During recovery phase of pernicious anaemia

Ideopathic thrombocytopenic purpura

In the elderly this condition has a chronic and fluctuating course. The platelet count is usually below 60×10^9 per litre. Megakaryocytes in bone marrow are reduced but in some may be increased. In these individuals there is little budding of platelets. Bleeding time is prolonged, and there is impaired prothrombin consumption and thromboplastin generation but, however, coagulation is normal. In some cases antibodies may be detected. Although some respond to corticosteroids, others may require splenectomy.

Causes of secondary thrombocytopenia
> — Bone marrow toxins
> — Drugs: sedormid, quinidine, quinine, sulphonamide, tolbutamide, chlorpropamide, digoxin, insulin, cimetidine, paracetamol
> — Chronic leukaemia
> — Pernicious anaemia
> — Neoplasm
> — Infection

MULTIPLE MYELOMA

> — A malignant disorder which is characterized by proliferation of a single clone of plasma cells. Although the peak incidence lies between 50–65 years it can occur in the older elderly. Clinical features include
> - Bone pain
> - Recurrent chest infections due to impaired immunoglobulins
> - Symptoms of anaemia
> - Symptoms of hypercalcaemia
> - Symptoms due to hyperviscosity
> - Root pain or spinal cord compression due to vertebral involvement
> - Peripheral neuropathy
> - Symptoms of acute renal failure due to deposition of protein in tubules, plasma cell infiltration and amyloidosis. The latter, which may produce nephrotic syndrome, is seen in approximately 10–25% of cases
> — The blood picture usually reveals anaemia, which can be normochromic, normocytic, leucoerythroblastic or macrocytic, with rouleaux formation. Platelet count may be reduced and ESR is often over 100 mm in the first hour. Bone marrow reveals excess of plasma cells and associated with this there is the presence of abnormal monoclonal protein, which in 50% of patients is of IgG type. Bence Jones protein, which is made of light (K or gamma) chains, is excreted in the urine in about 50% of patients. This type of protein, however, can also be found in patients with Waldenstrom's macroglobulinaemia and in cases of carcinoma with bony secondaries. Radiological examination of the skeleton may reveal osteolytic lesions in the spine, pelvis, skull or ribs. Despite the osteolytic lesions, the large

majority of patients, unlike those with bony metastases from other tumours, have normal serum alkaline phosphatase.
— Prognosis depends on age and tumour mass (large mass is indicated by haemoglobin of less than 8.5 g/dl, serum calcium greater than 2.68 mmol/l and serum IgG greater than 70 g/l, and the presence of osteolytic lesions).

Management
— Intermittent 4-day courses of melphalan and prednisolone or cyclophosphamide
— Radiotherapy to relieve bone pain
— Transfusion for severe cases

BENIGN MONOCLONAL GAMMOPATHY

This is present in about 6% of elderly over 80 years and in 14% in the group older than 90 years. Unlike multiple myeloma these patients do not have symptoms, and their IgG concentration, haemoglobin and ESR are normal and the marrow contains less than 9% plasma cells. Although it is regarded as a benign condition, it probably represents one end of a spectrum and the patient should be followed up regularly.

WALDENSTROM'S MACROGLOBULINAEMIA

This is a disease of the elderly, with the average age of the patient being 60 years. Two-thirds of patients are males and the hallmark of the condition is the presence of monoclonal IgM paraprotein produced by a clone of immature B-cell lymphocytes.
Clinical features include
— Fatigue
— Weakness
— Haemorrhages
— Weight loss
— Neurological disturbances
— Visual disturbances
— Thrombosis
— Hepatomegaly in 38%
— Splenomegaly in 37%
— Ocular changes in 37%
— Lymphadenopathy in 37%
— Haematological abnormalities in 20%
— Purpura in 16%
— Congestive heart failure in 4%
— Bence Jones protein in the urine

Treatment

Similar to that of multiple myeloma except plasmaphoresis may be used in cases of hyperviscosity syndrome.

BIBLIOGRAPHY

Antin J H, Rosenthall D J 1985 Acute leukaemia, myelodysplasia and lymphoma. In: Freedman M C (ed) Clinics in Geriatric Medicine. Saunders, Philadelphia

Bennet J M, Catovsky D, Daniel M T et al 1982 Proposals for the classification of the myelodysplastic syndrome. British Journal of Haematology 51: 189–199

Breedveld F C, Bieger R, Van Wermeskerken R K A 1981 The clinical significance of macrocytosis. Acta Medica Scandinavica 209: 319–322

Crawford J, Eye M K, Cohen H J 1981 Evaluation of monoclonal gammopathies in the 'well' elderly. American Journal of Medicine 82: 39–45

Editorial 1985 Waldenstrom's macroglobulinaemia. Lancet, 2: 311–312.

Strobach R C, Anderson S K, Doll D C, Ringenberg A C 1988 The value of the physical examination in the diagnosis of anaemia, correlation of the physical findings and the haemoglobin concentration. Archives of Internal Medicine 148: 831–832

15. THYROID GLAND DISORDERS

AGE-RELATED CHANGES

— With age there is a decrease in size of the follicles in the gland. This is associated with an increase in the number of microscopic and macroscopic nodules and an increase in connective tissue

— Studies on physiology have suggested a fall in iodine clearance (which is related to the loss of renal nephrons) and reduction in the rate of turnover of thyroxine, resulting in increase in half-life of thyroxine. However, the serum levels of T_4 and T_3 are usually not significantly affected by age, unless an illness is present in the elderly. Measurement of TSH levels have produced conflicting results. While some studies have demonstrated an increased percentage of elderly persons with raised TSH, others have shown no difference with age. TSH response to TRH has been noted to be blunted in some of the normal elderly, therefore caution is advised when interpreting the data from TRH test

THYROID DISEASE IN THE ELDERLY

The prevalence of thyroid disease increases with age and the elderly often present atypically, making biochemical confirmation of the disease mandatory; but the interpretation of thyroid function tests in the elderly is fraught with pitfalls. Abnormal thyroid function tests can be caused by thyroid disease, non-endocrine disease or concomitant drug therapy such as phenytoin, salicylates, oestrogen, non-steroidal anti-inflammatory agents and beta-blockers. Although these drugs interfere with T_4 binding and affect the value of total T_4, they do not affect the levels of free T_4 and T_3.

'Sick euthyroid syndrome'

The common cause of abnormal thyroid function tests in euthyroid individuals. In a variety of acute illnesses the T_3 production is impaired, resulting in a low T_3 level, and eventually there is a tendency for total T_4 level to fall too. However, along with the reduction in total T_4 level there is also a fall in T_4 binding globulin which results in increased availability of the unbound free T_4. Thus sick patients commonly have a low T_4 and a low T_3 on routine screening. This can be distinguished from true primary hypothyroidism by the absence of a rise in TSH. True hypothyroidism in the elderly ill patient is demonstrated by a low T_4 and a high TSH.

Subclinical hypothyroidism

— This is characterized by a T_4 at the lower end of the normal range and a moderately raised TSH. It is said to be present in 5% of the population, with a prevalence reaching 15% in women over 60 years. There is controversy as to the cause and management of this condition. Some maintain that it represents preclinical disease which if untreated will progress to true hypothyroidism, whereas others feel that it is the result of a 'sluggish' gland being able to maintain an adequate production of T_4 under the influence of increased amounts of TSH. Certainly subtle abnormalities of myocardial contractibility have been noted which reverse with thyroxine treatment in these individuals.

— A raised TSH in the presence of a low normal T_4 usually occurs in one of three situations
   1. After radioactive iodine treatment
   2. After thyroidectomy
   3. In presence of thyroid antibodies

— In the case of (1) and (2) this is usually a transient phenomenon. Thyroid function tests should be monitored monthly. If T_4 rises and the TSH returns to normal range, no further action is required. If T_4 falls and TSH rises and the patient is becoming clinically hypothyroid, then replacement therapy should be started. If the patient remains clinically euthyroid and thyroid function tests do not change, annual review is all that is necessary

— Patients with thyroid antibodies are particularly at risk of developing hypothyroidism. Therefore, if such a patient is noted to have a low normal T_4 and a moderately raised TSH with a high titre of anti-microsomal antibodies, they should be monitored carefully as progression to hypothyroidism in these patients is very likely

HYPOTHYROIDISM

The commonest cause of hypothyroidism is auto-immune thyroiditis; as
the incidence of auto-immune disease increases with age, this tends to be
a disease of the older age group and, as one might expect, women
predominate. It is a diagnosis which is easily missed because of its
insidious onset, and often symptoms such as tiredness, slowing up, etc.,
are attributed to ageing by the patient and the doctor.

Clinical features

Thyroid hormone deficiency affects all systems. Thus the patient may
complain of dry skin, hair loss, lassitude, constipation, cold intolerance
and weight increase despite anorexia.

On examination there may be evidence of other auto-immune disease
such as vitiligo or rheumatoid arthritis. The patient classically has
coarsening of facial features, puffiness of the face and eyes, loss of hair,
particularly at the lateral aspect of the eyebrows, and puffiness of the
hands and feet. The skin may be yellow due to carotinaemia and
patients may be noted to have bradycardia. Neurological examination
may reveal slow relaxation of tendon jerks. Effusions into serous
cavities, i.e. pleura, pericardium and abdominal cavity, are common, if
looked for, although they rarely cause complications. Untreated
hypothyroidism in the elderly can progress to confusion, psychosis and
even coma, and myxoedema coma may be precipitated by hypothermia.

Investigations

Diagnosis is confirmed by the finding of a low T_4 in the presence of a
raised TSH. The TRH test is usually unnecessary unless hypothalamic or
pituitary disease is suspected. Anaemia is common in patients with
hypothyroidism. This can be either normochromic, normocytic or
macrocytic. The latter may be secondary to pernicious anaemia but can
also be a direct result of the hypothyroidism. Forty-one per cent of
hypothyroid patients who do not have B_{12} deficiency have macrocytosis,
compared with the expected incidence of 9% in the elderly population.
An ECG usually shows bradycardia and small voltage complexes.
Pericardial effusions are often small and posterior, but if large may be
seen on a postero-anterior or a lateral chest X-ray. The effusion is
usually asymptomatic and requires no treatment other than that for
hypothyroidism.

Management

Replacement therapy should be instituted extremely carefully in the
elderly. Thyroxine should be started in a dose of 0.025 mg/day and
increased by 0.025 mg increments every month until the correct
replacement dose is reached. This is monitored by measuring T_4 and
TSH. Generally speaking, young adults require 2 μg/kg daily; the
elderly, however, require slightly less than this. The suggested dose is

1.8 $\mu g/kg$ per day but even this may be too much for the majority of the hypothyroid elderly.

Screening

The reported prevalence of hypothyroidism varies from 0.5 to 2.4% among the elderly. In view of this it has been advocated that screening should be carried out on all elderly. This is, however, probably unnecessary. Screening is, however, likely to yield a significant pick-up rate in the following groups

- Elderly women
- Those with past history of Grave's disease, those who have had treatment with radioactive iodine and those who have had thyroidectomy
- Those with thyroid antibodies (especially microsomal)
- Those with other auto-immune disease(s)
- Those with macrocytosis
- Those with increased prolactin levels

HYPERTHYROIDISM

The main causes of hyperthyroidism in old age are multinodular goitre, Plummer's disease, Grave's disease, thyroiditis, and ectopic hormone production by tumour and iodine.

Clinical features

The diagnosis of hyperthyroidism is more difficult in the elderly because not only are there fewer findings but the significance of those present may not be appreciated. The classical signs and symptoms, like tremor, nervousness, goitre with a bruit and exophthalmos, may be absent in the elderly. The patient may present with muscle weakness (proximal) with cramps, weight loss, atrial fibrillation with or without heart failure, diarrhoea, confusion or atypically with 'apathetic thyrotoxicosis', in which he or she complains of lethargy, depression and weight loss. The diagnosis can be confirmed by elevated T_4 level. In early thyrotoxicosis or more rarely in the presence of an autonomous nodule, the T_4 may be normal and only the T_3 is elevated. If there is doubt about the diagnosis, TRH test should be performed. This reveals a flat or absent response in thyrotoxicosis. However, it must be remembered that an impaired response can be obtained in euthyroid individuals in certain circumstances.

Management

- The thyrotoxic patient should initially be rendered euthyroid using anti-thyroid drugs such as carbimazole 45 mg/day. The concurrent use of beta-blockers, which is often advocated, is of little value and can prove to be dangerous in the elderly.
- Once euthyroid the patient should be offered radioactive

iodine (^{131}I) as this has the advantage of avoiding long-term oral therapy, is cheap and can be given on an out-patient basis. The disadvantage of this mode of therapy is its associated increased incidence of hypothyroidism. The risk is related to the dose of ^{131}I used. In view of this, long-term folllow-up of these patients is essential.

— Surgery is the treatment of choice if the thyrotoxicosis is associated with a large goitre producing pressure symptoms. If the patient refuses surgery or radioactive iodine treatment then anti-thyroid drugs should be continued on a long-term basis.

BIBLIOGRAPHY

Davis P J, Davis F B 1984 Hypothyroidism in the elderly. Comprehensive Therapy 10: 17–23

Editorial 1987 Subclinical hypothyroidism. Journal of the American Medical Association 258: 246–247

Falkenberg M, Kagedal B, Norr A 1983 Screening of an elderly female population for hypo- and hyperthyroidism by use of a thyroid hormone panel. Acta Medica Scandinavica 214: 361–365

Gambert S R, Tsitouras P D 1985 Effect of age on thyroid physiology and function. Journal of the American Geriatrics Society 33: 360–365

Levin R M 1987. Thyrotoxicosis in the elderly. Journal of the American Geriatrics Society 35: 587–589

Rosenthal M J, Sanchez C J 1985 Thyroid disease in the elderly: Missed diagnosis or over diagnosis. Western Journal of Medicine 143: 643–647

Rosenthal M J, Hunt W C, Garry P J, Goodwin J S 1987 Thyroid failure in the elderly: Microsomal antibodies as discriminant for therapy. Journal of the American Geriatrics Society 258: 209–213

Spaulding S V 1987 Age and the thyroid. In: Sackton B (ed) Endocrinology and ageing. Saunders, Philadelphia

16. DIABETES MELLITUS

— It is well known that glucose tolerance tends to deteriorate with increasing age. Although the exact cause of glucose intolerance is not clear, it has been shown to be associated with abnormalities of insulin secretion and/or action. The average 2-hour plasma glucose in the glucose tolerance test rises by approximately 0.5 mmol/l per decade after 50 years of age, and fasting levels by 0.06 mmol/l

— The hyperglycaemia of ageing is now regarded as of pathological significance, since it is associated with increase in glycosylated haemoglobin as well as with increased macrovascular disease, particularly coronary heart disease

Prevalence

— The occurrence of diabetes mellitus increases with age. The majority of the patients have type 2 diabetes, although some of the younger patients on insulin grow into old age and may present with either acute or chronic complications of the disease. The prevalence of diabetes mellitus in those aged 65 and over is three times that for below 65 years. Two-thirds of diabetic patients in hospital are over 65 years

— Type 2 diabetes is thought to be secondary to decreased insulin secretion and/or release, increased resistance to insulin and a decreased number of insulin receptors. It is thought that underlying genetic susceptibility plays a large part in these individuals

Presentation

— Often silent, and the patient is discovered as having diabetes only on routine blood or urine testing. Some patients, however, present with mild to moderate acute symptoms of weight loss, weakness, polydipsia, polyuria and polyphagia. Latter symptoms of course may be triggered by simple infection. Occasionally an elderly person may present with coma, seizure or focal neurological signs related to development of hyperosmolar non-ketotic diabetic coma.

— Younger diabetics who grow old may present with onset of microvascular or macrovascular complications.

Management

— It is a commonly held belief that type 2 diabetes mellitus is a less serious disease than insulin-dependent diabetes; however, this is far from the truth. Patients with type 2 diabetes are at just as much risk, if not more, of developing complications as those with type 1. In young diabetics there is enough evidence linking good diabetic control with decreased evidence of complications to justify for striving for near-perfect glycaemic control. In cases of an old or frail diabetic, one must weigh the possible benefits of improved control against disadvantages of severe disruption to their life-style. However, this does not mean that the elderly diabetic should be abandoned, and we should not try to achieve normoglycaemia; neither of course does it mean that complications should not be, where possible, prevented or treated.

Diet

— The mainstay of treatment in both type 1 and type 2 diabetes. The importance of sticking to the diet should be discussed not only with the patient but also with other members of the family or carers involved in providing food for that particular patient. Advice should be geared not only in terms of calories but also to decrease fat intake and increase the fibre in the diet in order to achieve a smoother blood sugar control. Patients should be given diet treatment for at least 2 months, provided they are not ketotic before hypoglycaemic agents are commenced

— In addition to diet, the elderly should be advised about the benefits of regular exercise, which not only improves glucose tolerance but also increases the utilization of calories and thereby leads to reduction in weight

Drugs

— Hypoglycaemic agents used fall into two groups
  • Sulphonylureas
  • Biguanides

— Sulphonylureas are a group of drugs which stimulate the release of insulin and potentiate its action peripherally. Short-acting agents such as tolbutamide are the drugs of choice for the elderly, since long-acting agents can lead to prolonged hypoglycaemia. If possible the sulphonylureas should not be used in the obese elderly as the hypoglycaemic effect induces hunger, which inevitably causes increased food intake leading to further increase in weight, worsening of diabetic control and a subsequent increase in dosage of sulphonylurea, thus creating a vicious circle

— The only biguanide in use is metformin. This is used particularly in those who require weight reduction as it has malabsorptive effect and induces anorexia. Unfortunately, sometimes it can be associated with unacceptable side effects, particularly nausea and diarrhoea
— Insulin is rarely required in the newly discovered diabetic, unless of course maximum doses of oral hypoglycaemic agents and diet have failed to control the hyperglycaemia
— In cases of insulin-dependent diabetics who have grown old one has to remember that their insulin requirement may decrease with ageing, therefore dosage may have to be adjusted accordingly
— Monitoring of diabetes can be carried out by most elderly diabetics, who can be taught to test their own urine. If, however, they are unable to do so then a health visitor or district nurse should be asked to test their post-prandial urine and/or blood by BM sticks

COMPLICATIONS OF DIABETES

Vascular disease

Both type 1 and type 2 diabetics have an increased susceptibility to vascular disease. The main physiological features of these complications are progressive narrowing of the lumen of both the small and large vessels and abnormal leakage of protein from the circulation. The main vascular complications which lead to increased morbidity and mortality among diabetics include coronary heart disease, cerebrovascular disease and peripheral arterial disease.

Diabetic feet

— Vascular complications, particularly involving the feet, are often compounded by the coexisting neuropathy. Both sensory neuropathy and autonomic neuropathy exacerbate the ulceration of feet in diabetics. Autonomic neuropathy causes dilatation of the arteriovenous shunts, thus leading to increased blood flow, which in turn diverts blood from the smaller vessels and the capillary nutrient circulation. This factor leads to relative distal ischaemia, rendering the foot more susceptible to forces of weight bearing and predisposing the foot to ulceration. Sensory neuropathy also makes the foot more vulnerable, particularly at pressure points commonly under the head of the first metatarsal bone. It increases the risk of damage from burns from hot-water bottles or by sitting too close to the fire or from pressure from ill-fitting shoes. Motor neuropathy can also contribute to the development of foot ulceration as it leads to atrophy of the intrinsic foot muscles and alteration of the shape of the foot, thus leading to undue pressure on some areas of the skin

— In view of this, and the presence of microthrombi in the small blood vessels, it is important that regular inspection of feet is carried out. Infections should be treated seriously and the toe-nails looked after by a chiropodist, particularly if the elderly have poor vision. Patients should also be advised about daily cleaning, with particular care to drying the areas between the toes

Ocular complications

— Ocular complications are present in many diabetics at the time of diagnosis. The patient, however, may not be aware of the visual loss even when it is severe. In view of this, regular checks on visual acuity are mandatory

— Amongst type 2 diabetics, proliferative retinopathy is less common and background retinopathy with maculopathy is much more likely to be seen. Visual loss in these patients is secondary to macular oedema or the presence of hard exudates in the macular region

— Patients with proliferative retinopathy do well with photocoagulation. Although it does not improve visual acuity it does prevent further deterioration. In addition to vascular complications in the eye, diabetics are also prone to cataract and glaucoma, which should be looked for and treated in the usual manner

Neuropathy

— The type of neuropathies that may be noted in diabetics include
  • Distal sensory plus sensorimotor neuropathy
  • Painful neuropathy
  • Mononeuritis
  • Mononeuritis multiplex
  • Plexus damage
  • Reticulopathy
  • Autonomic neuropathy

— Prevalence of neuropathy is greater in type 2 diabetics, and mononeuritis multiplex and amyotrophy are much more common in the elderly. Mononeuritis multiplex is a painful asymmetric neuropathy which may occur in patients previously undiagnosed as having diabetes mellitus. The pain, which is burning and severe, often starts in the hip and spreads to the knee. It tends to be more severe at night and is often associated with atrophy of the pelvic girdle and thigh muscles. Sphincter involvement may occur. Recovery may take months or even years

Diabetic amyotrophy

This is again seen more commonly in elderly men. It usually presents with progressive and painful weakness in the muscles of the pelvic girdle and sometimes associated with mild sensory changes. Usually the condition is self-limiting and resolves spontaneously in 6–12 months.

Autonomic neuropathy

The presence of autonomic neuropathy may be indicated by diarrhoea, postural hypotension, gustatory sweating, persistent tachycardia, intermittent vomiting and neurogenic bladder. The diarrhoea is usually intermittent and the patient may have several nocturnal exacerbations, which can lead to faecal incontinence. The presence of autonomic neuropathy can be assessed by simple objective tests, such as heart rate response to Valsalva manoeuvre, heart rate (R–R interval) variation during deep breathing, immediate heart rate response to standing, blood pressure response to standing and to sustained hand grip.

Nephropathy

Diabetic nephropathy, although more common amongst insulin-dependent diabetics, can present in elderly with type 2 diabetes. Proteinuria is the earliest sign of nephropathy. If renal function is impaired, risk factors such as hypertension and infection should be treated vigorously. The rate of progress of disease is best followed by measuring serum creatinine concentration. Recent data also suggest that the proteinuria could be reduced by good diabetic control, as well as with the use of angiotensin converting enzyme inhibitors or beta-blockers, which modify abnormal renal haemodynamics.

Urinary tract infection/papillary necrosis

— Urinary tract infection is common in both type 1 and type 2 diabetics and this can lead to renal papillary necrosis. Approximately 50% of patients with this complication are over the age of 65 years and one-third do not present with the classical symptoms and signs of loin pain and fever
— Prevention of renal papillary necrosis is by aggressive treatment of urinary tract infection. However, if it does

occur, renal function can be stabilized by continuous
antibiotic treatment

Hyperosmolar non-ketotic diabetic coma

— This is predominantly an acute complication encountered in
middle-aged and elderly patients, and is associated with very
high mortality. In some patients it is precipitated by factors
such as infection or myocardial infarction. Drugs such as
propanolol and thiazides have also been implicated in the
production of the coma. The patient has often been unwell
for several days prior to presentation, which in some can be
non-specific

— On examination the patient may be comatose, extremely
dehydrated and very ill. There is usually cardiovascular
collapse and incipient or established renal failure.
Laboratory tests confirm marked hyperglycaemia, usually
>50 mmol/l, increased plasma osmolality, hypernatraemia
and raised plasma urea. Bicarbonate and pH estimations
are, however, normal. Urinalysis may show heavy glycosuria
but ketones are usually absent. Treatment of this medical
emergency consists of correcting fluid and electrolyte
abnormalities, administration of insulin and treatment of the
underlying cause

BIBLIOGRAPHY

Bates A 1986 Diabetes in old age. Practical Diabetes 3: 120–123
Grenfell A, Watkins P J 1986 Clinical diabetic nephropathy: Natural history and
complications. Clinics in Endocrinology and Metabolism 15: 783–805
Lipson L G (editor) 1986 Diabetes mellitus in the elderly: Proceedings of a symposium.
Americal Journal of Medicine 80: 1–67
Morley J E, Mooradian A D, Rosenthal M J, Kaiser F E 1987 Diabetes mellitus in elderly
patients: Is it different? American Journal of Medicine 83: 533–544
Reaven G M, Reaven E P 1985 Age, glucose intolerance and non-insulin dependent diabetes
mellitus. Journal of the American Geriatrics Society 33: 286–290
Tattersal R B 1984 Diabetes in the elderly: A neglected area. Diabetologia 27: 167–173

17. ELECTROLYTE DISTURBANCES

— With increasing age there is a decrease in total body water, a fall in extracellular fluid and a tendency for serum potassium to rise, particularly in men. Serum sodium, however, shows no change apart from a small increase at the time of menopause
— The haemostatic mechanisms governing water and electrolyte balance are the same in the elderly as in young adults. However, these mechanisms are less efficient in the elderly and are readily upset. The age-related changes in glomerular filtration rate and the kidney's ability to conserve sodium and concentrate urine do not themselves produce electrolyte disturbances but do make the elderly more susceptible to developing them

HYPERNATRAEMIA

Causes

— Hypernatraemia, which may be defined as serum sodium of >145 mmol/l and osmolality of more than 290 mosmol/kg, has a stated incidence of about 1.1%. Although there are many heterogeneous causes the common contributory factors in the elderly are dehydration and infection
— Dehydration can result not only from increased fluid loss but also from decreased fluid intake, which may be secondary to poor mobility or confusion
— Infection can lead to dehydration, not only because it may lead to reduced intake but also because it may increase insensible loss due to tachypnoea, fever, increased catabolism, progressive obtundation and impaired thirst
— Less common causes of hypernatraemia in the elderly are hyperosmolar non-ketotic coma and nephrogenic diabetes mellitus. The latter not only results from pituitary lesions but also from diverse conditions such as myeloma, obstructive uropathy, hypercalcaemia, amyloidosis, potassium deficiency

and drugs, e.g. lithium, amphotericin, colchicine and demeclocycline

Clinical features

These can be non-specific and may include malaise and weakness. Thirst, however, is not always present or prominent. In severe hypernatraemia the patient may become comatose, with muscular rigidity and fits.

Treatment

Dependent on the factors producing hypernatraemia. Dehydration, which is a major factor in the majority of elderly patients with hypernatraemia, should be treated by fluid replacement. This should be achieved, if possible, orally or via a fine-bore nasogastric tube. If, however, this is not possible because of the patient's mental or physical state, then fluid should be replaced by IV route. Each patient should be treated vigorously, as the reported mortality from hypernatraemia ranges from 46 to 70%.

HYPONATRAEMIA

— This is a commonly encountered electrolyte disturbance seen in a high proportion of acutely ill elderly admitted to hospital. It is defined as serum sodium of less than 130 mmol/l. In about 50% of cases it is iatrogenic and the major factor responsible is diuretic therapy. Like hypernatraemia, it is associated with increased mortality and must be taken seriously
— A low serum sodium does not necessarily mean sodium depletion, and hyponatraemia can be of three types

Type 1 hyponatraemia

Total body sodium is depleted and extracellular fluid volume diminished. It is usually seen when there is excess sodium loss
— Excess loss via kidneys
  • Diuretic therapy
  • Mineralocorticoid deficiency
    – Addison's disease
    – Hypoaldosteronism
  • Chronic salt wasting
    – Chronic pyelonephritis
    – Analgesic nephropathy
    – After relief of obstruction
  • Diabetes mellitus
— Excess loss via gastrointestinal tract
  • Prolonged vomiting
  • Diarrhoea

- Ileus
- Fistulae
— Excess loss via skin
  - Excessive sweating
  - Burns

Clinical features
Usually non-specific and include confusion, lassitude, nausea, headache and muscle cramps. Postural hypotension is common and hands and feet may be cold and cyanosed. Those patients with very low sodium may exhibit neurological symptoms and signs, and these include convulsions, coma and Cheyne–Stokes respiration.

Treatment
Isotonic saline, usually given IV. In order to avoid fluid overload, urine output should be carefully monitored with a CVP line inserted to measure the venous pressure.

Type 2 hyponatraemia

Serum sodium is low, although total body sodium is increased, as is the extracellular fluid compartment. It is commonly seen in conditions where there is increased circulating aldosterone, such as heart failure, or in hypoalbuminaemic states, such as nephrotic syndrome. In these individuals, although the extracellular fluid volume is increased, there is decrease in the effective blood volume and this reduces glomerular filtration rate. The decrease in the effective blood volume also stimulates the production of ADH, which tends to exacerbate salt and water retention.

Clinical features
Clinical features are those of the underlying disease. Unlike type 1 hyponatraemia, oedema is always present. In those with severe hyponatraemia, i.e. sodium < 125 mmol/l, neurological symptoms such as confusion, muscle twitching and fits may develop.

Treatment
Treatment is directed at the underlying disease or cause. Salt and water should be restricted. In the presence of hyperaldosteronism, aldosterone antagonists, such as spironolactone should be used. In hypoalbuminaemic states plasma protein infusion may be helpful. One must remember that even in the presence of generalized oedema diuretics should be used cautiously as they may cause a further reduction in circulating volume and thereby exacerbate the electrolyte disturbance.

Type 3 hyponatraemia

Both total body sodium and extracellular fluid volume are normal, but ADH secretion is inappropriately increased.

Causes of increased ADH secretion
- — Lung disease
  - Infection
  - Tuberculosis
  - Neoplasm
  - Lung abscess
- — CNS disease
  - Stroke
  - Head injury
  - Tumour
  - Meningitis
  - Encephalitis
  - Subdural haematoma
  - Subarachnoid haemorrhage
- — Myxoedema
- — Alcohol
- — Drugs

Diagnosis is supported by low serum sodium, low plasma osmolality, inappropriately high urine osmolality (hypertonic urine) and persistently increased urinary excretion of sodium. The naturesis noted in some patients with inappropriate ADH secretion may be related to the high secretion of atrial naturetic factor (ANF).

Clinical features
Usually non-specific and symptoms and signs are those of the underlying condition.

Treatment
Treatment is of the underlying condition. Fluid, however, should be restricted to 500 ml daily and, if the hyponatraemia is symptomatic, demeclocycline is the drug of choice. In severely ill patients, however, hypertonic saline infusion may have to be given to correct the abnormality.

HYPERKALAEMIA

Causes
The commonest cause of hyperkalaemia in the elderly is potassium-sparing diuretics, particularly in those in whom renal function is already impaired. Other causes, which include factors which lead to spurious elevation of potassium, are
- — Diuretic therapy with potassium-sparing diuretic
- — Acute renal failure
- — Addison's disease
- — Hypoaldosteronism
- — Acidosis
- — Tissue necrosis
- — Haemolysis

Clinical features

May be absent until cardiac arrest occurs. Non-specific weakness and confusion are, however, often seen. ECG may show peaked T-waves, loss of P-waves and widening of QRS complexes. In severe cases it may lead to ventricular fibrillation or standstill.

Treatment

— Urgent treatment is required if potassium is more than 6.5 mmol/l. As cardiac arrest can be precipitated by rough handling, patients should be nursed in a high-dependency unit and monitored while 10% calcium gluconate or dextrose/insulin infusion or sodium bicarbonate is given IV. Sufficient amount of 10% calcium gluconate should be given to cause a return to normal of peaked T-waves

— If the above emergency measures fail, dialysis should be considered

— Oral ion exchange resins such as calcium resonium, which is given orally or by retention enema, are useful but do not act immediately.

HYPOKALAEMIA

Causes

Hypokalaemia is a common abnormality noted in about one patient in 20 taking diuretics. The other causes which may lead to hypokalaemia are loss of potassium from the renal tract or from the gastrointestinal tract

— Renal loss
  - Recovery from obstruction
  - Renal tubular acidosis
  - Hyperaldosteronism
  - Cushing's disease
  - Diuretics
  - Ketoacidosis
— Gastrointestinal loss
  - Vomiting
  - Diarrhoea
  - Purgative abuse
  - Fistulae
  - Villous adenoma
  - Ileus
  - Uterosigmoid anastamosis
— Decreased dietary intake
— Loss from skin via excess sweating

Clinical features

Non-specific; may include apathy, weakness and confusion.

Hypokalaemia can, however, also lead to paralytic ileus, features of renal tubular damage or to cardiac conduction defects, particularly in those with myocardial ischaemia or on digoxin therapy. ECG changes which may be noted include tall U-wave and prolongation of PR interval.

Treatment

Aims at treating the underlying cause as well as giving potassium supplements; the latter should be given orally wherever possible.

BIBLIOGRAPHY

Cogan E, Debieve M-F, Pepersack T, Abramow M 1988 Natriuresis and atrial natriuretic factor secretion during inappropriate antidiuresis. American Journal of Medicine 84: 409–418

Jaffrey L, Martin A 1981 Malignant hyperkalaemia after amiloride/hydrochlorothiazide treatment. Lancet 1: 272

Lye M D W 1985 The milieu interieur and ageing. In: Brocklehurst J C (ed) Textbook of geriatric medicine and gerontology (3rd edn). Churchill Livingstone, Edinburgh pp. 201–229

Snyder N A, Feigel D W, Arief A I 1987 Hypernatraemia in elderly patients: A heterogeneous, morbid and iatrogenic entity. Annals of Internal Medicine 107: 309–319

Surinderam S G, Mankikar G D 1983 Hyponatraemia in the elderly. Age and Ageing 12: 17–18

18. NUTRITION

Changes in the nutritional status of the elderly are brought about by alterations in their socio-economic circumstances, which often occur about the time of retirement, by the increasing incidence of disease and disability which lead to changes in dietary intake, absorption and metabolism of nutrients, and in some cases by a number of drugs which are prescribed for the elderly. All these changes, both environmental and medical, become more marked in the second half of the eighth decade.

Metabolic rate

— The total energy production per square metre of body surface falls progressively with advancing age. The average decrement is about 12 cal/m^2 per hour for each year between the ages of 20 and 90 years. This fall is believed to be due to loss of metabolizing tissue with age, since animal experiments show there is no decrease in oxygen uptake of tissue slices, homogenates or isolated mitochondria taken from various organs

— The total energy production per 24 hours is the sum of basal energy production and that required for daily activities. The calories required for activities fall more than the basal calories, especially in very old individuals. There is fairly close agreement between caloric intakes and energy expenditure at all ages. The reduction in energy metabolism in old age is a reflection of tissue loss and to a greater extent, particularly in the very old, of reduction in physical activity. The limited capacity for exercise is due to the increasing incidence of disease and disability after the age of 75, and the main causes are degenerative joint disease and disorders of the respiratory and cardiovascular systems

— The importance of exercise is clearly seen in a study by Durnin et al (1966) of elderly farmers. The lowest energy output was 2200 kcal/day and the highest was 4200 kcal/day. Thus in a group of men from the same socio-economic background engaged in the same occupation, one man could expend twice as much energy as another

7777 NUTRITION 159

Recommended intakes of nutrients

— There are many 'standards' for energy and nutrient intakes which have been formulated in various countries. The recommendations for the UK have been published by the DHSS (1969 and 1979a). The values for elderly people are shown in Tables 18.1 and 18.2
— The values for energy are similar to those recommended by the FAO/WHO, except the UK values for elderly women are considerably higher. The values for the elderly, however, are based on estimates of the average rate at which activities decline. Thus they take into account the diminution in energy expenditure associated with the increasing incidence of physical infirmity in old age. There are many individuals whose activities are well maintained in old age and whose calorie intakes are much greater than the recommended values

Table 18.1 Recommended daily intakes of energy and nutrients for elderly people in the UK

	Men		Women	
	65–74	over 75	55–74	over 75
Energy (kcal)	2350	2100	2050	1900
Protein (g)	59	53	51	48
Thiamine (mg)	0.9	0.8	0.8	0.7
Riboflavin (mg)	1.7	1.7	1.3	1.3
Nicotinic acid (mg)	18	18	15	15

From DHSS (1979a).

Table 18.2 Recommended daily nutrient intakes which do not change with age

	Men over 65	Women over 55
Calcium (mg)	500	500
Iron (mg)	10	10
Ascorbic acid (mg)	30	30
Vitamin A (μg retinol)	750	750
Vitamin D (μg cholecalciferol)	2.5	2.5

MALNUTRITION

Definition
Malnutrition may be defined as a disturbance of form or function due to lack of (or excess of) calories or of one or more nutrients (DHSS 1972).

Obesity, which is included in this definition is a problem in old age and after the age of 75 it is much more common in women than in men, but it usually results from long-standing faulty eating habits. Undernutrition, on the other hand, results from environmental and physical factors which usually affect people in later life.

Prevalence

The results of a DHSS (1972) survey of the elderly based on random samples of old people living at home in six areas of the UK showed a prevalence of malnutrition of 3%. This includes protein–calorie malnutrition, iron deficiency and vitamin deficiencies. When the subjects were followed up 5 years later the proportion with malnutrition had increased to 7% and the prevalence was found to be twice as high in those over the age of 80 compared with those aged 70–79 years (DHSS 1979b).

Causes

There are two main groups of factors leading to nutritional deficiencies in the elderly and these are shown in Table 18.3.

Table 18.3 Causes of nutritional deficiencies

Primary	Secondary
Ignorance	Impaired appetite
Social isolation	Masticatory inefficiency
Physical disability	Malabsorption
Mental disturbance	Alcoholism
Iatrogenic	Drugs
Poverty	Increased requirements

Ignorance
The King Edward's Hospital Fund survey (Exton-Smith and Stanton 1965) showed that ignorance of the basic facts of nutrition is common in elderly women. Their views had often been formulated many years ago, often in childhood, when dietary habits had been dictated by financial stringency. It is likely that in men ignorance is even more important, especially in the recently widowed who may have to fend for themselves for the first time and they may have little idea of what constitutes a balanced diet.

Social isolation
For many old people living alone in social isolation there is a loss of interest in the preparation and cooking of food. What food is eaten is usually taken in the form of snacks. Dietary surveys show that nutrition is much better in those who have a number of outside interests and in those who eat at clubs in the company of others.

Physical disabilities
Hemiplegia, arthritis, impairment of vision and other physical disorders

can lead to difficulty in getting and preparing food. The housebound living alone are particularly vulnerable unless they have adequate support from others.

Mental disturbances
Surveys show that the unmet medical, nursing and social needs are greatest in those old people with psychiatric disorders. Malnutrition occurs in dementia, but for a demented old person to be maintained at home care must be provided by others and nutrition is often adequate. Depressive illness is probably a more important cause since it often leads to a disinclination to obtain, to cook and even in severe cases to eat food.

Iatrogenic
A badly planned dietary regime may lead to malnutrition, especially when it is continued longer than necessary. For example, cases of scurvy have been reported in patients having a gastric diet for peptic ulcer since this may be deficient in vitamin C.

Poverty
The food eaten by pensioners is often dull, monotonous and tasteless. Old people who are able to supplement their income from savings or from part-time earnings have a better diet than those whose sole financial means is the retirement pension.

Impairment of appetite
Both transitory and long-continued impairment of appetite are common in old age. The time taken for recovery of appetite following an infection or a surgical operation is longer than in the younger person. Frank malnutrition may be precipitated in a patient whose nutrition was previously only marginally adequate.

Inefficient mastication
A poor state of dentition may favour especially soft foods consisting mainly of carbohydrate, while more nutritious foods requiring mastication are avoided. One study showed that subjects with few remaining teeth but no dentures performed about as well as those wearing dentures of indifferent quality.

Malabsorption
Mild degrees of malabsorption are not uncommon in the elderly. This may be due to small bowel ischaemia, gluten sensitivity or other causes (see p. 114). The absorption of fat and fat-soluble vitamins and of folic acid and vitamin B_{12} is mainly affected.

Alcohol and drugs
When alcohol intake is excessive, energy needs may be derived mainly from this source and the intake of other nutrients may be curtailed. Folic acid metabolism is impaired in some alcoholics and megablastic anaemia occurs. Many drugs impair appetite, for example the cytotoxic agents used in the treatment of cancer patients, who may already be malnourished. Other examples of drugs interfering with nutrition are impairment of folic acid metabolism in those taking barbiturates and

anticonvulsants; enzyme induction in those taking anticonvulsant drugs can also lead to vitamin D deficiency.

Increased requirements

Negative nitrogen balance and the breakdown of tissue protein can occur in patients who are immobilized in bed for long periods, in those who suffer from long-continued pyrexia, and as a result of extensive bed sores with the loss of protein-rich fluid (see below). The extent to which this can be reversed by supplementation with high intake of protein is uncertain.

Vulnerable groups

The housebound

— A combination of primary and secondary factors often operate together to produce malnutrition. Sometimes the factors are interrelated; for example, limited mobility, loneliness, social isolation and depression are all found in housebound old people and make them especially liable to malnutrition when they are receiving insufficient care from others

— The housebound have been shown to have nutrient intakes which are substantially lower than those of active people matched for age (Exton-Smith et al 1972). Since about 10% of the elderly population are housebound, i.e about three-quarters of a million old people in the UK, this section of the population represents the largest single group vulnerable to malnutrition. Thus disability in old age not only affects the mode of living but it also has an adverse effect on nutritional status

Risk factors

Eleven risk factors (both medical and environmental) predisposing to malnutrition (seven significant risk factors are shown in Fig. 18.1) were identified in the second survey of the elderly population conducted by the DHSS (1979b)

— Living alone
— No regular cooked meals
— Receipt of supplementary benefit
— Social classes IV and V
— Reduced mental test score
— Depression
— Chronic bronchitis and emphysema
— Gastrectomy
— Poor dentition
— Difficulty in swallowing
— Housebound state

There was a highly significant difference ($p<0.001$) in the distribution of risk factors between the malnourished and the non-malnourished; thus

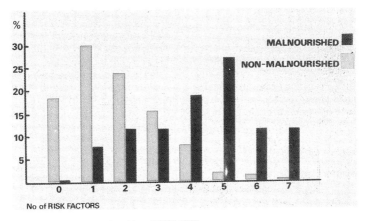

Fig. 18.1 Risk factors in malnutrition. DHSS 1979b

27% of the malnourished had five of these risk factors compared with 2% of the non-malnourished.

Protein–energy malnutrition

Protein metabolism

— The total amount of protein in the body declines with age. The body composition of subjects between the ages of 25 and 75 years has been studied on a longitudinal basis by Forbes & Reina (1970). Using [40]K counting it was found that the lean body mass (LBM) declines progressively after the age of 25, whereas body fat increases, so that the total body weight fails to reveal the continuous decrease in LBM. Men weighing approximately 75 kg at the age of 25 have an average LBM of 61 kg and a fat content of 13 kg, but by the age of 65 the LBM has declined by 12 kg (20%) and the body fat has risen by 15 kg (120%) without any marked change in total body weight

— It has been calculated that a dietary allowance of 0.35 g of protein/kg body weight is adequate to maintain nitrogen balance in young subjects under ideal conditions (Munro 1972); but for older subjects under less artificial conditions the need is nearer 0.6 g/kg body weight. The recommended intakes for the UK (DHSS 1969) are considerably higher than this and are calculated on the basis that protein should contribute 10% of the total energy requirements. For the normal utilization of dietary protein sufficient energy must

be available, and the protein–energy relationship is more important than the absolute amount of protein. Particularly in the elderly account must be taken of the quality and the amino acid composition of dietary proteins; thus the needs for the essential amino acids methionine and lysine, which cannot be synthesized, rise sharply after the age of 50 years
— Serum albumin concentration decreases with advancing age. The total albumin pool is 20% lower in healthy elderly subjects compared with young controls. Since homeostasis of serum albumin levels is maintained by a mechanism in the liver which is sensitive to osmotic pressure, it has been suggested that a decline in sensitivity of this mechanism is responsible for the fall in serum albumin

Prevalence

— In the DHSS survey (1972) a search was made in all subjects having low energy intakes for malnutrition. Of the 88 subjects in this category (men with intakes of less than 1500 kcal/day and women with intakes of less than 1200 kcal/day) 8 were thought to have protein – calorie malnutrition on the basis of the clinical assessment and a serum pseudocholinesterase activity of less than 150 units
— In the whole sample 13% had serum albumin concentrations of less than 3.5 g/100 ml. Forty per cent of these subjects with low serum albumin levels had oedema. The additional effects of stress of non-nutritional disease (mainly congestive cardiac failure) was in part responsible

Effects of illness

— The significance of subclinical malnutrition, including protein deficiency, is difficult to assess. It may, however, be of greater importance in the elderly than at other ages since homeostatic mechanisms are often impaired. Stress due to a variety of diseases which are common in old age may upset the precarious physiological balance
— The total body protein turnover in a group of ill elderly in-patients has been measured using a tracer dose of [^{15}N]glycine, (Phillips 1983). In comparison with normal elderly controls the ill subjects had significantly higher total body nitrogen flux, protein synthesis and breakdown rates, but significantly lower plasma albumin. This increased protein turnover in spite of reduced muscle mass in the ill subjects appears to be due to the effects of tissue trauma and inflammation. It is not known, however, whether the failure to maintain the body pool of albumin in ill old people can be influenced by increased dietary intake. Also, it has yet to be established if a higher intake of protein and other nutrients would confer benefits on the older individual

who is in a state of subclinical malnutrition and enable him
to resist more effectively the effects of stress due to
non-nutritional disease

ANAEMIA AND IRON DEFICIENCY

The normal levels of haemoglobin (Hb) and erythrocytes (RBC) as
defined by WHO study groups (WHO 1968) are: for men, 13 g/100 ml
and 4.7 ×10 per mm^2, and for women 12 g per 100 ml and 4.0×10 per
mm^2 respectively. Normal old people are not anaemic, and Hb and RBC
levels below these limits should not be ascribed to old age.

Clinical features
— Lack of iron leads to microcytic, hypochromic anaemia,
which if sufficiently severe produces tiredness, lack of
energy, breathlessness on exertion and palpitations. A
milder degree of anaemia, especially if the development is
slow, gives rise to few symptoms because of compensatory
mechanisms which lead to more efficient release of oxygen
from the haemoglobin
— Various tissue changes occur in iron deficiency; the most
characteristic is koilonychia, with spoon-shaped deformity of
the nails. Patients often complain of a sore tongue which
becomes smooth and redder than normal due to atrophy of
the papillae. The Plummer–Vinson syndrome resulting from
a web of mucosa in the post-cricoid region is rare. But lack
of acid secretion in the stomach is common and the gastric
mucosa may show atrophic or inflammatory changes
— Severe anaemia with typical manifestations is rarely due to
poor dietary intake alone; in such cases there are nearly
always other causes of blood loss, for example
gastrointestinal haemorrhage

Prevalence
— In the DHSS (1972) report the overall prevalence of
anaemia in the elderly population was 7.3% and was about
the same in the two sexes. The only factors for which a
significant correlation with Hb was found were mode of
living and serum iron concentration. Those living alone
more often had anaemia (9%) compared with those who
lived with their spouse or relatives (6%); this difference was
significant ($p<0.01$)
— Iron deficiency was the sole cause of anaemia in only
12.9%. Iron deficiency associated with subnormal serum
folate levels was found in 22.6% of anaemic subjects, and
iron deficiency with subnormal vitamin B$_6$ levels in 8.1% of

anaemic subjects. In a further 20% of anaemic subjects all three serum levels were subnormal. One-third of old people with anaemia had a normal serum iron concentration and in nearly half of these (14.6%) the serum iron, folate, vitamin B_6 and vitamin B_{12} levels were normal
— Investigations carried out in elderly patients in hospital show a much higher frequency of anaemia. In a survey coordinated by the DHSS (1972) anaemia was found in 27% of males and 32% of females. The major cause is haemorrhage, particularly from the gastrointestinal tract

Significance of iron deficiency

An investigation of 45 clinically healthy persons (aged 57–71 years) in a double-blind study showed that the group given ferrous fumarate (60 mg iron) for 3 months had an increase in physical work capacity as measured with a bicycle ergometer (Ericsson 1972). A decrease in total iron-binding capacity (TIBC) occurred only when it was initially high and only in the group treated with iron. Elwood & Hughes (1970), however, were not able to demonstrate any benefits from iron supplementation in improving symptoms and psychomotor performance in younger subjects.

VITAMIN B COMPLEX DEFICIENCY

Clinical manifestations

Changes in the mucous membranes and lips include
— Cheilosis: red, denuded, often scaly epithelium at the line of closure of the lips
— Angular stomatitis: greyish white, sodden and swollen epithelium, progressing to fissuring, radiating outwards from the corners of the mouth
— Nasolabial seborrhoea: enlarged follicles around the sides of the nose, and plugged with sebaceous material
— Glossitis: bare, red, smooth tongue with loss of filiform papillae, sometimes associated with fissuring and enlargement of the fungiform papillae

Development of changes

Five stages in the development of vitamin deficiency disease based on observations of human thiamine deficiency have been proposed (Brin 1968). The overt disease is not manifest until stage 4. During the physiological stage the three symptoms are loss of appetite, general malaise and increased irritability — all common complaints due to many other causes in the elderly.

In stages 4 and 5, thiamine deficiency leads to cardiac and neurological manifestations including bradycardia, cardiac enlargement, oedema, peripheral neuropathy, mental confusion and ophthalmoplegia. Wernicke's encephalopathy is almost certainly due to thiamine deficiency. The clinical features include diplopia and nystagmus, progressing to ophthalmoplegia and the mental changes of Korsakoff's psychosis: loss of memory, confabulation, disorientation and hallucinations.

Significance of deficiencies

— The nutritional status for vitamin B complex in the elderly population has been investigated in several surveys, the most comprehensive being that conducted by the DHSS (1972). Up to one-quarter of the subjects had biochemical evidence of deficiency of thiamine or riboflavin, but the number with overt clinical deficiency was very small

— The true significance of marginal deficiency is at present unknown, but laboratory tests may serve to identify those individuals who might benefit from vitamin supplementation to prevent the development of acute deficiency disease.

— Thurnham et al (1979) have shown that old people who eat vitamin-fortified breakfast cereals have better riboflavin and thiamine status than those not eating these cereals. Again this marginal deficiency was only detected on the basis of biochemical tests

— Older & Dickerson (1982) have shown that elderly patients undergoing hip replacement and other operations for fracture of the femoral neck had temporary postoperative thiamine deficiency lasting up to 14 days. Those who were most confused after the operation had biochemical evidence of the most marked deficiency

Folate deficiency

Clinical manifestations

Folate deficiency causes a general disturbance in which various tissues and organs are involved, but the main clinical findings are anaemia, and changes in the nervous system and in the mucous membrane of the tongue.

— The anaemia is megaloblastic, characterized by abnormal nucleated red cell precursors (megaloblasts) in the bone marrow and macrocytes in the peripheral blood. There is an associated leucopenia and hypersegmentation of the neutrophils; the number of platelets may be reduced

— In patients with chronic neurological diseases, especially peripheral neuropathy, the changes are more often due to folate deficiency than to vitamin B_{12} deficiency. Mental changes may precede the anaemia; they are non-specific and include mild confusion, depression, apathy and cognitive impairment

— The tongue may be sore and the surface red due to acute glossitis, but it is more commonly smooth, shiny and atrophic

Causes

The main causes of folate deficiency in the elderly are inadequate intake, malabsorption, increased utilization and impaired effectiveness.

— Dietary inadequacy is an important cause of deficiency. A mixed diet contains 500–800 μg/day, but as it is mainly in the reduced form the folate is readily destroyed by sunlight, oxidation and cooking. The minimum requirement is 50–100 μg per day, but many times this amount may be required if there is increased utilization

— Absorption of folate occurs in the upper small intestine and it may be impaired in gluten enteropathy and other conditions producing the malabsorption syndrome

— Folate requirements increase when cell turnover increases, e.g. in haemolytic anaemia, myeloproliferative syndromes, carcinoma, myeloma and in some chronic inflammatory conditions such as tuberculosis and Crohn's disease

— The effectiveness of available folate is impaired under certain conditions, e.g. vitamin C deficiency inhibits folate coenzymes and in scurvy-impaired folate metabolism is one of the causes of megaloblastic anaemia. Various drugs, including methotrexate, anticonvulsants and trimethoprim, interfere with folate metabolism

Folate status in the elderly

— The extent of anaemia and of folate deficiency has been reported in the DHSS survey (1972) of the elderly population (see p. 164). There is also a reservoir of old people in the population who suffer from folate deficiency without being significantly anaemic. To what extent these deficiency states have an adverse effect on health is uncertain

— A much higher frequency of folate deficiency has been reported in patients admitted to geriatric departments. A dietary origin was suspected in many of the patients; folate deficiency is more common in disabled people who are unable to look after themselves. A statistically significant relationship has been found between organic brain disease and low serum and red cell folate levels

ASCORBIC ACID DEFICIENCY

Scurvy has almost disappeared from our population, but it is occasionally seen in the elderly, especially in men. It is sometimes referred to as 'bachelor's scurvy', but it is more appropriately called widower's scurvy as it most often occurs in men who after the death of the spouse have to fend for themselves.

Clinical features

— Manifestations include swelling and bleeding of the gums (not in edentulous individuals), weakness, anaemia, extensive haemorrhages in the skin of the legs and arms ('sheet haemorrhages') and sometimes haemorrhages at other sites.

— Anaemia is common in scurvy. It is usually normocytic or macrocytic with normoblastic or macronormoblastic erythropoiesis; but cases of true megaloblastic anaemia have been reported. It is often multifactorial in origin: haemolysis, bleeding, dietary deficiency of iron and derangement of red cell metabolism

— Mental changes are probably common in scurvy. Depression and personality changes occur in experimentally induced ascorbic acid deficiency

— Wound healing may be delayed. The administration of vitamin C may promote the healing of pressure sores by increasing collagen formation

Vitamin C status of old people

— Although signs of overt deficiency are rare, the body stores of vitamin C in many old people are diminished. Low levels of leucocyte ascorbic acid (LAA) have been reported in many studies. The levels are lower in the elderly than in younger subjects, lower in winter than in summer, lower in men than in women, and smokers have lower LAA levels than non-smokers

— Diminished LAA levels are found in institutionalized old people. They have been attributed to the effects of cooking of such foods as potatoes, the delay in the delivery of the meal to the recipient and an inadequacy of fruit and fruit juices. Similar factors may be responsible for the inferior vitamin C status of old people receiving meals-on-wheels, which are cooked in institutions and kept hot in containers

— In a study of the elderly population in Edinburgh it has been shown that LAA levels are significantly higher in July to December compared with those when blood samples were taken during the rest of the year. Vitamin C intake correlated with LAA level and it was found that LAA levels increased in parallel with, but lagged behind, seasonal increases in vitamin C intakes

Significance of low tissue stores

— The Edinburgh and other surveys have shown that there is a significant number of old people whose ascorbic acid intake is less than 10 mg/day, which is known to be the amount required to prevent or cure scurvy. The recommended allowance of 30 mg/day takes into account the considerable individual variation in requirements and the extra needs due to stress. Although a high proportion of elderly people are consuming less than 30 mg/day the majority will not suffer any ill-effects

— Surveys have also shown that about one-quarter of the men and 10% of the women have LAA levels of less than 15 $\mu g/10^9$ WBC, which is taken as the lower limit of normal for the elderly. The higher proportion of men with deficiency is in keeping with the clinical finding that scurvy is more prone to occur in men than in women

— A study of elderly patients in hospital in Cornwall showed that mortality could be related to LAA levels, but subsequent investigation revealed that the severity of illness influenced the tissue stores of vitamin C as well as the mortality. Moreover, the administration of vitamin C failed to produce an increase in LAA in many of the patients, nor did it influence mortality

VITAMIN D DEFICIENCY

In the elderly this is usually multifactorial in origin. The main clinical manifestation is osteamalacia, but it is also found in some patients with fracture of the femoral neck.

Clinical manifestations
— The clinical features of osteomalacia are described on p. 185. The possible clinical indications are shown below and the diagnosis should be suspected when these conditions are present
  • Vague and generalized pain
  • Low backache
  • Muscle weakness and stiffness
  • Waddling gait
  • Skeletal deformity
  • Bone tenderness
  • Malabsorption states
  • Long confinement indoors
  • Malnutrition
— Vitamin D deficiency is also of clinical significance in the absence of the usual features of osteomalaci. Studies in the MRC Mineral Metabolism in Leeds (Aaron et al 1974) have shown by histological examination that 20–30% of women with fracture of the proximal femur and about 40% of men have histological evidence of osteomalacia. The proportion with abnormal osteoid-covered surfaces varied with the season

Vitamin D status of the elderly population

— Studies using radio-stereo assay of 25-hydroxycholecalciferol (25-OHD) have shown seasonal variations in both the old and the young. Summer sunlight is probably the chief determinant of vitamin D nutrition in Britain
— In summer 25-OHD correlates with amount of sunlight exposure and is independent of the vitamin D content of the diet, whereas in winter the levels correlate with dietary intake and the amount of sunlight exposure the previous summer
— The effects of age on 25-OHD levels have been examined by Dattani et al (1984). In both sexes there was a linear decline between the ages of 65 and 90 years; the winter levels were lower than those in summer, and both were lower in women than in men. The summer levels declined more rapidly than the winter levels and by the age of 90 in each sex the summer levels equalled the winter levels. This study clearly shows the effects of limitation of sunlight exposure due to the diminished outdoor activity in very old people

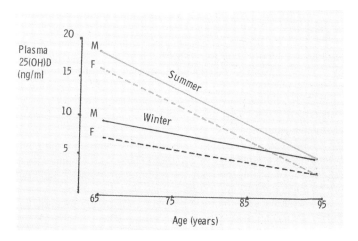

Fig. 18.2 Decline in plasma 25-OHD with age. From Dattani et al (1984)

PREVENTION OF MALNUTRITION

The factors can be identified in most forms of nutritional deficiency in the elderly. Although malnutrition can occur in isolation, it is more often associated with other unmet medical and social needs.

Vulnerable groups

Old people especially at risk are the socially isolated, those with physical disorders including impairment of the special senses which contribute to isolation, the recently bereaved, very old men living alone, and those with mental disorders. It would be unrealistic to apply preventive measures to all old people since the majority will not develop malnutrition. Thus the groups at risk must be identified. The largest group at risk is the housebound, who constitute about 10% of old people living in their homes. The majority of housebound are already known to the health and social services.

Assessment of nutritional status

The primary medical care team is responsible for the assessment of those especially at risk. The assessment should ideally be carried out by a dietitian; his or her skills will also be required in giving advice when the diet is found to be inadequate. When clinical malnutrition is suspected the general practitioner can often confirm the diagnosis using appropriate biochemical and haematological investigations.

Club meals and meals-on-wheels

When old people eat at clubs in the company of others, an improvement in nutrition can often be achieved. Many find it is convenient to have a club meal since there is no shopping, cooking or washing-up to be done. To make an effective contribution to the total dietary intake at least four club meals a week should be eaten.

About 1.5% of old people receive meals-on-wheels, but the real need is probably much greater than this. The meals service is usually provided by the WRVS, and regular visits to the homes of housebound old people do much to prevent social isolation. The domiciliary meal, as in the case of the club meal, should be as nutritious as possible, since the recipient tends to regard it as the main meal of the day.

Nutrient supplementation

The best means of promoting food nutrition is by improving the quality, and in some cases the quantity, of the diet. Thus when vitamin C intake is inadequate it can be improved by the addition of oranges, tomatoes, blackcurrant juice and rose-hip syrup.

The very low intake of vitamin D and lack of exposure to sunlight must lead to a consideration of supplementation. This could be done by the fortification of milk, which is a procedure adopted in the United States. In the first instance the distribution of fortified milk might best be restricted to housebound old people.

BIBLIOGRAPHY

Aaron J E, Gallagher J C, Anderson J, Stasiak L, Longton E B, Nordin B E C, Nicholson M 1974 Frequency of osteomalacia and osteoporosis in fractures of the proximal femur. Lancet 1: 229–233

Brin M 1968 Biochemical methods and findings in US surveys. In: Exton-Smith A N, Scott
    D L (eds) Vitamins in the elderly. Wright, Bristol
Dattani J, Exton-Smith A N, Stephen J M L 1984 Vitamin D status of the elderly in relation
    to age and exposure to sunlight. Human Nutrition: Clinical Nutrition 38C: 131–137
DHSS 1969 Recommended intakes of nutrients for the United Kingdom. Report on Public
    Health and Medical Subjects No 120 HMSO, London
DHSS 1972 A nutritional survey of the elderly. Report on Public Health and Medical Subjects
    No 3, HMSO, London
DHSS 1979a Recommended daily amounts of food energy and nutrients for groups of people
    in the United Kingdom. Report on Health and Social Subjects No 15 HMSO, London
DHSS 1979b Nutrition and health in old age. Report on Health and Social Subjects No 16
    HMSO, London
Durnin J V G A, Lonergan M E, Wheatcroft J J et al 1966 The energy expenditure and food
    intake of middle-aged and elderly farmers. Proceedings of the VIIth International Congress
    of Nutrition, Hamburg
Elwood P C, Hughes D 1970 Clinical trial of iron therapy on psychomotor function in
    anaemic women. British Medical Journal 3: 254–255
Ericsson P 1972 Iron metabolism in the elderly. In: Carlson L A (ed) Nutrition in old age.
    Almquist & Wiksell, Uppsala
Exton-Smith A N, Stanton B R, 1965 Report on an investigation of the diet of elderly women
    living alone. King Edward's Hospital Fund, London
Exton-Smith A N, Stanton B R, Windsor A C M 1972 Nutrition of housebound old people.
    King Edward's Hospital Fund, London
FAO/WHO 1973 Expert committee on energy and protein. FAO–WHO, Geneva
Forbes G B, Reina J C 1970 Adult lean body mass declines with age; Some longitudinal
    observations. Metabolism 19: 653–663
Munro H M 1972 Protein metabolism and requirements in ageing. In: Carlson L A (ed)
    Nutrition in old age Almquist & Wiksell, Uppsala
Older M W J, Dickerson J W T 1982 Thiamine and the elderly orthopaedic patient. Age and
    Ageing 11: 101–107
Phillips P 1983 Protein in the elderly: A comparison between ill patients and elderly controls.
    Human Nutrition: Clinical Nutrition 37C: 339–344
Thurnham D I, Hassan F M, Powers H J 1979 Effects of riboflavin deficiency on erythrocytes.
    In: Taylor T G (ed) Importance of vitamins to human health. MTP Press, Lancaster
WHO 1968 Nutritional anaemias. Technical Report Series, WHO No 405

19. NEUROPATHIES AND MYOPATHIES

PERIPHERAL NEUROPATHIES

In the elderly the common causes are diabetes mellitus, alcoholism, malignancy and drug toxicity. In many cases, in spite of intensive investigation, a cause cannot be found. The disorder of function can affect the sensory, motor and autonomic nerves.

Diabetes mellitus

— The most frequent manifestation is a sensory neuropathy with pain in the limbs, especially at night. Loss of vibration, light touch and proprioception in the legs can usually be detected. There may also be loss of pupillary reflexes
— Involvement of the autonomic nervous system causes intermittent nocturnal diarrhoea, impaired temperature regulation and orthostatic hypotension (see Ch. 10); involvement of the sacral outflow can produce voiding problems due to a hypotonic bladder (see p. 257)
— The most important motor manifestation is diabetic amyotrophy producing asymmetrical painful muscle weakness in the legs, particularly in the quadriceps. Unilateral or bilateral foot drop may occur
— The neurological complications of diabetes tend to occur in long-standing, poorly controlled diabetes. It is often mild in degree and may not require hypoglycaemic agents for its control. When treatment is required insulin is to be preferred rather than oral agents

Alcoholism

— The patient with alcoholic peripheral neuropathy complains of painful paraesthesiae in the feet and hands, painful muscle cramps and difficulty in maintaining balance. Wrist drop can occur owing to flaccid paralysis of the wrist extensors. The calves are often tender and the ankle jerks absent. Autonomic neuropathy may occur but it is less common

than in diabetes
— Peripheral neuropathy is usually a feature of Wernicke's encephalopathy; this is due to thiamine deficiency, most often associated with alcoholism. The salient features are ophthalmoplegia, nystagmus, ataxia, orthostatic hypotension and impairment of thermoregulation. Korsakoff's psychosis may be present, with loss of short-term memory and confabulation
— Treatment consists of the withdrawal of alcohol and the correction of nutritional deficiencies, especially thiamine. Any improvement in peripheral neuropathy is usually slow, as it is with mental disturbances in Korsakoff's psychosis. The response to thiamine administration in Wernicke's encephalopathy is often dramatic

Malignancy

— Peripheral neuropathy is a non-metastatic manifestation of several malignancies, notably oat-cell carcinoma of the bronchus, carcinoma of breast, ovary, stomach and the reticuloses.
Neurological signs may be sensory, motor, autonomic or mixed and may precede other clinical indications of the tumour
— Other non-metastatic features may be present, for example, myopathy and polymyositis. Symptoms may remit when the tumour is removed

Drug toxicity

Many drugs have been reported to cause peripheral neuropathy. Toxic effects are more common in the elderly owing to altered drug metabolism. Some of the causes are listed in Table 19.1.

Table 19.1 Agents causing peripheral neuropathy

Heavy metals and organic compounds	Drugs
Arsenic	Isoniazid
Lead	Ethambutol
Mercury	Nitrofurantoin
Gold	Vincristine
Thallium	Phenytoin
Lithium	Dapsone
Acrylamide	Chloroquine
Tri-orthocresyl phosphate	Hydralazine
Carbon disulphide	Metronidazole

Vitamin B$_{12}$ deficiency

— Peripheral neuropathy is sometimes an early feature of vitamin B$_{12}$ deficiency. Paraesthesiae occur in the feet and fingers — the patient may complain that the sheet feels rough, like a blanket. There may be peripheral cutaneous sensory loss and stabbing pains in the legs

— With the development of subacute combined degeneration of the cord there is loss of vibration (often to the level of the iliac crests), position sense and ankle and knee jerks; the plantar responses become extensor

— The response to treatment with vitamin B$_{12}$(cytamen) weekly is better for peripheral neuropathy than it is for subacute combined degeneration of the cord

DISEASES OF MUSCLE

Age changes

— Muscle power diminishes with age. Measurement of the strength of quadriceps contraction shows that power increases from the age of 10–14, to reach the highest level in the 20–29-year age group, remaining unchanged until 40–49 years and thereafter gradually declining. Hand-grip strength declines markedly with age and at 80 years it is about half that of 20-year-olds. Males at all ages have a stronger hand grip than females

— The decline in muscle strength with age is due to loss of muscle bulk, which in turn is paralleled by a reduction in the area of type II (fast twitch) muscle fibres. Training programmes in subjects over the age of 65 years have shown that it is possible to increase quadriceps strength by more than 20%, an increase which is comparable to that which can be attained in young adults. Moreover, a programme of exercises, in addition to improving muscle strength, increases type II muscle fibre area in the elderly and reverses type II fibre atrophy.

— Multiple aetiological factors are probably involved in the production of muscle weakness and wasting in old age. The most important appear to be due to changes in the central and peripheral nervous systems with fall-out in the anterior horn cells and reduction in the number of motor units. Muscle biopsy shows changes of chronic denervation, especially in the over-75s, when muscle wasting becomes accentuated. Immobility can certainly cause muscle weakness, particularly when it is due to painful and stiff joints leading to localized muscle atrophy; it is unlikely, however, that it is a primary cause of general muscle weakness in old age. Nutrition surveys of the elderly population have revealed a relationship between protein–calorie malnutrition and reduction in lean body mass. The suggestion that there is a causal relationship between muscle strength and dietary potassium intake has not been substantiated

MYOPATHIES

The commoner causes are

— Drugs, such as lithium, propranolol, atenolol, bumetanide, vincristine and cimetidine can cause an acute or subacute proximal myopathy. Large doses of corticosteroids lead to a similar myopathy, often associated with muscle pain

— Alcoholic myopathy with a rapid onset of muscle weakness and pain can occur a few days after an episode of heavy drinking in a chronic alcoholic. If alcohol can be withdrawn recovery usually occurs

— Non-metastatic carcinomatous myopathy with generalized muscle wasting occurs in most carcinomas, especially when the patient's nutritional status is affected. A proximal myopathy with weakness and wasting occurs in carcinoma of the bronchus, pancreas, gastrointestinal tract, breast and prostate

— Thyrotoxic myopathy consists most commonly of a proximal muscle weakness. The tendon reflexes are often brisk. Improvement usually occurs when the hyperthyroidism is treated

— Osteomalacia characteristically leads to proximal muscle weakness. The symptoms are a waddling gait produced by tilting the pelvis while walking in an attempt to raise the feet from the ground. There is often difficulty in rising from a chair and in climbing stairs. When the shoulder girdle muscles are involved the patient has difficulty in raising the arms above the head and performing such activities as brushing the hair. The muscle condition is painless, but pain may be due to fracture, pseudofracture or bone tenderness. Treatment with vitamin D is usually effective but the response is often slow, over a period of 3–6 months. Myopathy occurs in hyperparathyroidism when it is secondary to osteomalacia

— Hypokalaemia produces periodic muscle paralysis which tends to occur when the plasma potassium falls below 3 mmol/1. The likely causes are long continued use of diuretics, excessive purgation and protracted vomiting. An ancillary factor in the elderly is a low potassium intake

MYASTHENIA GRAVIS

An uncommon condition which occasionally occurs in the elderly. A myasthenic state, however, can accompany a non-metastatic carcinomatous myopathy, usually due to oat-cell carcinoma of the bronchus.

Clinical Features

Characteristically there is muscle weakness aggravated by exertion and improved by rest. Muscles predominantly affected are those supplied by the cranial nerves, and the weakness produces ptosis, diplopia, ophthalmoplegia, dysphonia and dysphagia. Weakness of the lower limbs occurs in 10–15% of cases.

Aetiology

There is strong evidence that myasthenia gravis is an auto-immune disease:

— Antinuclear antibodies, IgG, antibodies against acetylcholine receptors and antistriated muscle antibodies are found in a high proportion of cases, especially when thymoma is present
— There is also impaired T cell functioning and humoral immunity
— It is associated with other diseases which have an autoimmune basis, notably systemic lupus erythematosus, polymyositis and hyperthyroidism

The weakness and fatiguability in myasthenia is probably due to interference with neuromuscular transmission resulting from binding of antibody to post-junctional acetylcholine receptors.

Diagnosis

Can be confirmed by

— The response to Tensilon (edrophonium chloride). In the test 2 mg of Tensilon are given IV, followed by 8 mg if no improvement occurs within 1 min
— The finding of impaired responsiveness to repetitive nerve stimulation on the EMG

Treatment

Neuromuscular transmission can be improved by correcting the acetylcholine deficiency by the use of anticholinesterase drugs

— Neostigmine (15–30 mg at intervals throughout the day when maximum strength is needed) has a duration of action of 4 h. The use of the drug can be limited by powerful muscarinic side effects, which may require treatment with anticholinergic drugs simultaneously

— Pyridostigmine (30–120 mg at intervals throughout the day) has a slower action but longer duration and is less powerful. Side effects are minor

— Distigmine(5 mg daily before breakfast initially, increasing with care) has an even longer duration of action and is mainly used for those patients who are weak when getting up in the morning. A cholinergic crisis may occur due to accumulation.

The response to treatment in the myasthenic state associated with malignancy is poor, as is the response to the Tensilon test.

— Thymectomy is the treatment of choice. Improvement is often greater than from the use of anticholinesterase drugs, although the response in the elderly may be less marked

— Oral steroids are mainly used for patients who have failed to respond to thymectomy and to anticholinesterase drugs

— Drugs suppressing the immune system, such as cyclophosphamide, can be used when there has been little improvement on other therapy.

POLYMYOSITIS

Polymyositis is a rare inflammatory myopathy of uncertain cause, but an autoimmune basis is most likely. Cases have been reported in patients in their eighth decade.

Clinical features

— There is a progressive symmetrical muscle weakness of the proximal muscles of the limbs, of the neck and abdomen. The patient may have difficulty in getting in and out of a chair and on climbing stairs. Dysphagia and respiratory muscle weakness may occur. Involvement of the smooth muscle of the oesophagus produces hypomotility. Progression is variable, either constant or with relapses and remissions. Muscle contractures are seen in the later stages

— When polymyositis is associated with an erythematous skin rash the condition is known as dermatomyositis. The purple rash is located over the cheeks, neck, upper chest, the extensor surfaces of the knees and elbows and over the knuckles

— There is an association of polymyositis and dermatomyositis with malignancy, especially of the bronchus, breast, ovary, prostate and the gastrointestinal tract. They are sometimes a manifestation of reticuloses

Treatment
Patients with malignancy should have the tumour removed if possible. In the absence of malignancy steroids should be given: prednisolone 60 mg

daily. Maintenance doses should be adjusted according to the clinical
response which is usually slow. Azothioprine, methotrexate and
cyclophosphamide have also been used.

POLYMYALGIA RHEUMATICA

Polymyalgia rheumatica is a disorder of older people characterized by
aching pain and stiffness in the proximal muscles. The mean age of onset
in most reported series is 65–70 years.

Clinical features

— Characteristically the symptoms are diffuse, poorly localized
muscular pains around the shoulders and also in the lumbar
region, buttocks and thighs. The striking feature is severe
morning stiffness, particularly around the shoulders. When
the pelvic girdle muscles are involved the patient may have
difficulty in getting out of bed without assistance. The onset
is acute rather than gradual. In addition, there are
constitutional symptoms, malaise, depression, anorexia,
weight loss and low-grade fever

— Polymyalgia rheumatica forms part of a symptom complex
of giant cell arteritis. About 30% of patients have temporal
artery involvement. Typically the presentation is with
throbbing unilateral headache. The temporal arteries may be
swollen and tender along their course and extending into
the scalp, making it painful to brush the hair. In patients
with giant cell arteritis 50% experience visual disturbances at
some time due to involvement of the ophthalmic arteries.
When the arteries supplying the masticatory muscles are
affected the patient complains of claudication pain on
chewing

Diagnosis

— There are no specific diagnostic features of polymyalgia
rheumatica, but discriminant function analysis has identified
seven characteristics of value in diagnosis, (Bird et al 1979)
- Shoulder pain and stiffness bilaterally
- Onset of illness of <2 weeks duration
- Initial ESR >40 mm per hour
- Morning stiffness lasting >1 hour
- Age >65 years
- Depression and /or loss of weight
- Upper arm tenderness bilaterally

— The presence of three or more of these features makes the
diagnosis of polymyalgia rheumatica probable and a prompt
response within 2 weeks to prednisolone 10 mg daily
substantiates the diagnosis

— Although typically the ESR is raised often to levels of 100 mm/h or more there are cases of polymyalgia with giant cell arteritis confirmed by biopsy where the ESR is normal. Moreover, the range of ESR in healthy elderly people is 3–60 mm/h and it is therefore difficult to assess the significance of a raised ESR

Treatment

— Prednisolone should be given in the usual starting dose of 10 mg daily. After 2–3 weeks the dose can be reduced gradually. The development of arteritis after reduction of the dose requires the prompt initiation of high-dose therapy (prednisolone, 60 mg daily) to prevent such serious complications as visual loss.
— The patient should be followed up every 2–3 months during the first year and encouraged to report relapse or symptoms suggestive of cranial arteritis. The maintenance dose of prednisolone is rarely greater than 5 mg daily. The condition is self-limiting and it is uncommon for a relapse to occur after 3 years

CRAMP

Muscular cramps are common in the elderly and some 75% experience cramp. The usual clinical picture is of an individual who retires to bed at night free from symptoms and is awakened from sleep with severe pain in the calf. The calf muscles are contracted, hard and tender. The sufferer often gains relief by pressing the foot against the floor. The pain rarely lasts more than one minute but may be followed by muscle tenderness. Other sites may be involved, particularly the muscles of the sole of the foot and the big toe
— The majority of individuals who have cramp are in good health. There is, however, an association between cramp and arthritis of the hips and knees, varicose veins and a history of thrombophlebitis. Excessive muscular activity during the daytime is a factor favouring the development of cramp
— The essential mechanism is tetanic contraction of a group of muscle fibres. It may be precipitated by elongation or stretching of the fibres beyond a certain point. Sometimes the muscle stretching may be due to unconscious movements on awakening from sleep, or to sudden jerking movements in the legs in patients with arthritis of the knees. These influences and the fact that they tend to occur during rest following activity probably account for the nocturnal incidence of cramp
— Treatment is aimed at prevention of cramp. The two drugs

commonly used are quinine sulphate in a single dose of 200 mg at night and mephenesin 250–500 mg at night. It is difficult to assess the results of therapy because cramp may only occur infrequently, with long intervals between episodes

BIBLIOGRAPHY

Bird H A, Esselinckz A, Dixon A St J, Mowat A G, Wood P H N, 1979 An evaluation of criteria for polymyalgia rheumatica. Annals of the Rheumatic Diseases 38: 434–439
Dixon A StJ, Beardwell C, Kav C, Wanka J, Wong Y T, 1966 Polymyalgia rheumatica and temporal arteritis. Annals of the Rheumatic Diseases 25: 203–208

20. BONE DISEASES

AGE-RELATED CHANGES

With advancing years there is linear bone loss with respect to age, the loss being more rapid in women than men. The rate of loss in weight of bone is about 0.5–1% per annum in women after the menopause and in men from the age of 60 years. The loss affects the trabecular bone more than the cortical and on histology patients with post-menopausal spinal osteoporosis have trabecular bone of less than 14%, the normal for the elderly being 14–24%.

Though all women apparently lose bone after menopause, not all develop the degree of osteoporosis which results in fractures. The predisposing factors are probably a low initial mass, an accelerated rate of bone loss ('fast bone losers') or both.

OSTEOPOROSIS

Diminution of bone in which the bone is normally mineralized but the amount of bone in proportion to the volume of anatomical bone is reduced. It may result from increased bone resorption, reduced bone formation or both, and the causes are
- Immobilization
- Menopause
- Age-related (senile)
- Short stature and small bones
- Calcium deficiency
- Protein deficiency
- Vitamin D deficiency
- Vitamin C deficiency
- Fluoride deficiency
- Steroid excess (endogenous or exogenous)
- Rheumatoid arthritis
- Hyperparathyroidism
- Thyrotoxicosis
- Gastrectomy

— Alcoholism
— Smoking
— Liver disease
— Diabetes mellitus
— Heparin treatment

Clinical features

Symptoms in the elderly are variable. Some have no complaints, whereas others classically present with back pain which is variably associated with compression fracture of one or more vertebrae. The pain may be precipitated by stress but is usually self-limiting and disappears in 4–6 weeks. Other patients may present with fractures, loss of height, 'dowager's hump' deformity due to collapse of midthoracic vertebrae and fractures. Fractures involving the femur and the radius are common and about 30% of females with fractured neck of femur have osteoporosis, compared to 15% of males. The fractures occur not only because of osteoporosis but also because of increased tendency of the elderly to fall.

Investigations

— Biochemistry is essentially normal, although there may be increase in fasting calcium excretion in some women. Radiology reveals increased translucency, prominent vertical trabeculae, vertebral collapse, cod-fish vertebrae, widening of marrow cavity in long bones and fractures involving ribs, femur and radius. Unfortunately, these changes are only subjective

— Objective methods of measurement of cortical bone include photon absorption, neutron activation analysis (measurement of ^{49}Ca produced by neutron bombardment) and computed tomography. These methods can be used to measure changes with time, particularly to assess response to treatment

Treatment

— There is no simple treatment for osteoporosis that is universally acceptable. Various pharmaceutical substances either alone or in combination have been tried and all have been shown to produce some improvement in the cortical bone mass; these include oestrogens, calcium, Vitamin D, fluoride, calcitonin, stanozolol (an anabolic steroid) and cyclic regimen using a high-dose pulse of etidronate

— The dosages that have been tried either alone or in combination include
  • Stilboestrol, 1–3 mg/day
  • Ethinyloestradiol, 10–15 μg daily given every 3 weeks out of 4
  • Calcium, 1–1.5 g/day
  • Vitamin D, 1000 IU/day or 50 000 IU twice a week
  • 1,25-Dihydroxy-D, 0.25 μg/day

- Fluoride, 22.5–45 mg/day
- Calcitonin, 100 IU/day
- Stanozolol, 5 mg/day

— The post-menopausal bone loss in women can also be slowed down or prevented by the use of oestrogens and calcium supplements. However, these have to be started at the menopause and given for the rest of the natural life. It is this fact and the unwanted side effects, such as breast tenderness, nausea and irregular uterine bleeding, that make this measure unacceptable to the majority of the elderly and their doctors. In addition to oestrogen and calcium supplements, it is clear that a reasonable level of exercise can reduce the bone loss.

OSTEOMALACIA

Osteomalacia is a metabolic disease of bone characterized by deficient calcification of normal bone matrix. The estimated prevalence in the elderly population is about 3.7%. Histological examination reveals increased amount of osteoid, e.g. non-calcified matrix. It is a disease that is produced by lack of Vitamin D, which can result from many causes. However, in the elderly the aetiology is often multifactorial.

Causes
— Lack of sunlight
— Malabsorption
— Gastrectomy
— Liver disease including cholestasis
— Renal disease
— Drugs: barbiturates

Clinical features

Patients with osteomalacia may present with bone pain, bone tenderness, muscle weakness, general ill health, aches and pains and falls leading to immobility. Bone pain is common and can involve the chest, back, thighs and feet, and the pain is often made worse by stress. In some patients tenderness may be associated with pain. As the pain can be vague it may be misdiagnosed as being due to muscular rheumatism, arthritis or even disc disease. The muscular weakness mainly involves the proximal muscles and can lead to difficulty in getting out of a chair or climbing stairs and to, of course, waddling gait abnormality. Fractures associated with osteomalacia are common and one study has shown osteomalacia to be responsible for 20–30% of fractured neck of femur in women and about 40% of fractured neck of femur in men.

Investigations

— Investigations which may be useful in the diagnosis of osteomalacia include bone biochemistry, radiology, isotope bone scan and bone biopsy. Biochemistry typically reveals low or normal serum calcium, low serum inorganic phosphorus and raised serum alkaline phosphatase associated with low urinary calcium and low 25-hydroxycholecalciferol. Having said this, bone biochemistry can be completely normal in some patients with mild osteomalacia

— In patients with hypophosphataemic osteomalacia associated with carcinoma of the prostate the characteristic features are low serum phosphate associated with low renal phosphate threshold concentration, normal parathyroid hormone level, normal 25-hydroxy-D_3 and low 1,25-dihydroxy-D_3

— Radiological findings in osteomalacia are variable but the only diagnostic feature is the presence of Looser's zone or pseudo-fractures, which are bands of decalcification. The common sites where Looser's zones may occur are scapulae, pubic rami, the ribs, the neck of the humerus and the lesser trochanter of the femoral neck. In addition to the Looser's zones on radiology one may note wedge-shaped vertebrae, thicker trabeculae, subperiosteal reabsorption of phalanges due to secondary hyperparathyroidism and fractures, involving ribs and femur

— On isotope bone scanning the features which suggest the presence of osteomalacia include generalized increased uptake, focal uptake at the anterior ends of the ribs, focal uptake in the areas of Looser's zones, increased uptake in the mandible, increased uptake in the area of sternoclavicular joints giving a 'tie' sign and an 'absent kidney sign' on posterior view of abdomen reflecting reduced excretion of radiopharmaceutical agent and increased uptake by the skeleton. None of these features, unfortunately, is diagnostic but as the bone scanning is very sensitive it can suggest the presence of disease at the very early stages. Bone biopsy, of course, is the only way of confirming the diagnosis athough this can produce conflicting results as well. If, however, the patient is too frail or not willing to have investigations, then a trial of Vitamin D should be instigated

Treatment

Treatment of osteomalacia is vitamin D. This can be given orally or parenterally or by increasing the production of vitamin D by using ultraviolet light. As elderly patients tend to have low calcium in the diet, it is advisable to give them calcium with vitamin D. The preparations that can be used include calcium with vitamin D, BP tablets 1 bd, or calciferol given orally or parenterally (1000–1500 IU daily). In addition to treating the osteomalacia, the underlying condition producing it must be treated.

PAGET'S DISEASE OF THE BONE

Paget's disease of the bone is common in old age. It affects 2–4% of people over 60 years of age and 10% of the population over 85. It has a geographical distribution and is common in the UK, USA, Germany and France but is less common in the rest of Europe, Australia and New Zealand, and is rare in the Scandinavian countries as well as in Japan and Africa. In addition it tends to run in families.

As a condition it is characterized by a combination of excessive bone reabsorption and deposition. Both can result not only in deformity of the skeleton but also fractures. Although any bone can be involved, commonly affected bones are the skull, long bones, pelvis, sacrum and spine.

Clinical features

Like other metabolic bone diseases, symptoms of Paget's disease are variable. Patients may be asymptomatic or develop pain, bony deformities, fractures, neurological complications, cardiovascular complications and neoplastic changes in the areas affected by the disease. Neurological complications include involvement of cranial nerves (second, eighth, seventh and branches of the fifth), involvement of the cerebellum, obstruction to flow of CSF leading to internal hydrocephalus and spinal cord and nerve root compression. Cardiovascular complications include high-output heart failure but this is rare and tends to occur only in those with extensive disease. Those with extensive disease may also present with apathy and lethargy.

Investigations

Diagnosis can be made by bone biochemistry, which usually reveals markedly increased alkaline phosphatase with a normal calcium and phosphate, by radiology or isotope bone scanning or by bone biopsy.

Treatment

— The main aim of treatment of Paget's disease of bone is to alleviate the symptoms and to avoid the complications. Asymptomatic patients require no treatment. Those with intractable pain, neurological complications, heart failure or with extensive disease should be treated with calcitonin, which inhibits osteoclasts. Dosage should be 100 units daily for at least 6 months and after this the therapy should be adjusted according to activity of the disease

— In addition to calcitonin, diphosphanate (disodium etidronate, 200 mg/kg daily for 4–6 weeks), which can be taken by mouth, has been tried with some success.

Unfortunately, however, it has a tendency to produce bone demineralization in the elderly and therefore has to be used with caution. Lastly, cytotoxic agents like mithramycin have also been tried with some good effect.

METASTATIC BONE DISEASE

The skeleton is a very common site for metastases from sarcoma, and carcinoma of the breast, bronchus, prostate, thyroid and kidney.

Clinical features

— Metastases may be silent or produce bone pain, which is characteristically present at rest, wakes the patient at night, and responds poorly to simple analgesics. There may be bony swelling and deformity with local tenderness to percussion

— Compression of nerve roots, occurring with spinal metastases, causes referred pain, sensory disturbance, and weakness and wasting of innervated muscles

— Metastases may also present very acutely, with severe pain due to pathological fractures occurring without precipitating trauma, or with only very minor stress

— Bones most frequently involved are the vertebrae, proximal femur, pelvis, ribs, sternum and proximal humerus

— Hypercalcaemia, secondary to bone infiltration, may itself cause symptoms such as confusion, constipation, polyuria and abdominal pain

— In case of prostatic carcinoma hypophosphataemia may lead to the development of osteomalacia and therefore to symptoms of bone pain and muscle weakness. These symptoms respond to 1-α-hydroxy vitamin D with oestrogen

Investigations

— Radiological changes are absent in early metastatic disease, although radioisotope bone scan will show areas of increased uptake very early in the disease. The metastases may be sclerotic (as in carcinoma of the prostate and breast) or lytic (most other carcinomas and multiple myeloma). They are therefore seen on X-ray as areas of increased or reduced density

— The main biochemical abnormality is elevation of serum alkaline phosphatase, although this is by no means invariable. There may also be hypercalcaemia, which can occur in the absence of skeletal metastases, due to production of parathyroid-like peptide by the tumour

— Manifestations of disseminated malignancy include elevation of the ESR and a normochromic, normocytic anaemia

— Other abnormalities on investigation, reflecting the primary tumour, may of course be found

Treatment

— The presence of skeletal metastases (unless there is a single well-defined deposit) generally implies that the tumour is incurable, although some hormone-dependent tumours respond very well to chemotherapy, even when disseminated, with prolonged remissions, e.g. carcinoma of the breast may respond well to tamoxifen, and prostatic cancer may do very well on anti-androgens, such as stilboestrol or cyproterone acetate, with good relief from bone pain

— Non-steroidal anti-inflammatory agents, through their prostaglandin inhibition, often control metastatic bone pain better than simple analgesics, but severe pain requires opiate analgesia

— Steroids are very useful, both for their analgesic and euphoriant effect, and for treatment of hypercalcaemia

— Calcitonin is also useful in pain control, as well as having a calcium-lowering effect, but its use is limited by the intramuscular route of administration

— Radiotherapy gives good palliation, with relief of local bone pain and reduction in compression on surrounding structures, such as nerve roots

PRIMARY MALIGNANT BONE DISEASE

Chrondrosarcomas

Chrondrosarcomas are the commonest primary malignant bone tumours of later life. Most are located in the pelvic girdle, ribs and upper ends of the femur and humerus.

Clinical features
They present with bone pain, swelling and deformity. They are generally slow-growing and slow to recur.

Investigations
There are no biochemical abnormalities. X-ray shows bony destruction with areas of calcification.

Treatment
Radical excision is the treatment of choice.

Osteogenic sarcomas

These tumours generally occur between the ages of 10 and 40, but also occur in the elderly, secondary to Paget's disease. They usually arise in the distal femur and proximal tibia in young people, but in the elderly the site depends on the pattern of their Paget's disease.

Clinical features

Pain and swelling are the presenting features. An exacerbation of the pain of Paget's disease should arouse suspicion.

Investigations

Alkaline phosphatase may be raised, but there are no other biochemical abnormalities.

X-rays show bony destruction with lytic lesions, sometimes containing areas of abnormally dense bone, discontinuation in the surrounding cortex and periosteal reaction.

Treatment

— These are aggressive tumours, which metastasize early to the lungs and have a poor prognosis
— Combinations of intensive chemotherapy, radiotherapy and radical excision or amputation are necessary to try to control the tumour

---

OSTEOMYELITIS

Bacterial infection of bone may be direct, with infection introduced by trauma or surgery, or arising from a contiguous site of infection, of which the commonest is a neuropathic cutaneous ulcer, common in diabetic patients. Alternatively, spread may be haematogenous and this is often more difficult to diagnose. The commonest bony site of haematogenous infection is the vertebrae, which have cellular marrow and an abundant blood supply. Infection may spread between vertebrae by direct extension through the intervertebral disc or via communicating venous channels. Rarely, long bones at the extremities or the clavicles are involved.

ACUTE OSTEOMYELITIS

Clinical features

— Haematogenous osteomyelitis starts with a bacteraemia, from a urinary infection, distant soft tissue infection or endocarditis. However, the bacteraemic episode may be low-grade and not clinically apparent in the elderly
— The lumbar vertebrae are involved much more frequently than other parts of the vertebral column
— The onset of back pain and systemic signs of infection are frequently insidious and progressive. The pain is classically

constant, exacerbated by movement and unrelieved by rest or analgesia. Fever may be minimal or absent
— On examination of the spine, local tenderness over affected vertebrae is found, with reduced spinal movement and paravertebral muscle spasm

Investigations
— A high ESR is common, but the white count is often normal, or only mildly elevated
— Some patients may also have abnormal liver function tests and this may lead to an erroneous diagnosis of hepatitis or malignant liver disease. X-ray abnormalities are characteristic, but do not develop for several weeks. Soft tissue densities due to paravertebral abscesses may be visible and there is erosion of the subchondral bone, with narrowing of the intervertebral disc and bone destruction with sclerosis
— In early disease, before X-ray changes develop, radio-isotope bone scan will show areas of increased uptake, but these changes are non-specific
— Culture of the blood may reveal the organism and should be performed in all suspected cases, but the pick-up rate is disappointingly low
— Bone biopsy is usually necessary to confirm the diagnosis (malignant disease may look very similar on X-ray) and to isolate the organism. This is normally carried out by needle biopsy, under X-ray control, but open biopsy is occasionally undertaken
— *Staphylococcus aureus* is the commonest organism responsible for acute osteomylitis, but Gram-negative infections from the urinary tract also occur; polymicrobial infections, including anaerobic bacteriae, may result from a contiguous infection. Tuberculous and fungal osteomyelitis are uncommon. Culture of material from draining sinuses or ulcers is unreliable evidence of bone infection, as these areas may be colonized by skin bacteria, not present inside the bone

Treatment
— Appropriate IV antibiotics are given, after isolation of the organism, for 6–8 weeks
— Surgery is necessary to drain soft tissue abscesses and vertebral stabilization is performed only for unstable cervical spine disease
— Bed-rest is normally advocated in the early stages of treatment, but in the elderly rapid mobilization with analgesia and lumbar support may be more appropriate

CHRONIC OSTEOMYELITIS

Clinical features
This may follow acute bacterial osteomyelitis, or result from tuberculous infection. It tends to affect peripheral joints more often than the acute form. The main clinical feature is the chronic discharging sinus, and there is often little or no systemic disturbance and less pain than in acute disease.

Investigations
— The white count and ESR are unremarkable
— X-ray abnormalities are classical, with bone and disc destruction and evidence of new bone formation, with a periosteal reaction — known as the 'involucrum'

Treatment
— The mainstay of treatment is surgical, with debridement of necrotic bone and tissue, and elimination of dead space. Antibiotics alone are rarely effective, but should accompany surgical measures, and are usually given for at least 6 weeks, except in cases of tuberculosis when at least 6 months of anti-tuberculous treatment will be required
— If the osteomyelitis is associated with a prosthesis or other foreign body, this generally has to be removed
— In osteomyelitis associated with vascular insufficiency, and in severe chronic disease, amputation may be the only effective cure

BIBLIOGRAPHY

Campbell G A, Kemm J R, Hoskins D L, Boyd R V 1984 How common is osteomalacia in the elderly? Lancet 2: 386–388
Christiansen C (ed) 1987 Osteoporosis 1987: Cyclical etidronate for osteoporosis. International Symposium on Osteoporosis. Denmark
Christiansen C, Riis B J, Rodbro P 1987 Prediction of rapid bone loss in postmenopausal women. Lancet 2: 1105–1108
Drugs and Therapeutics Bulletin 1984 Osteoporosis and its treatment 22: 1–4
Hamdy R C 1981 Paget's disease of bone: Assessment and management. Fletcher, Norwich
Heath D A 1987 Treating Paget's disease. British Medical Journal 294: 1048–1050
Murphy P, Wright G, Rai G S 1985 Hypophosphataemic osteomalacia associated with prostatic carcinoma. British Medical Journal 290: 194
Preston C J, Yates A J P, Beneton M N C et al 1986 Effective short term treatment of Paget's disease with oral etidronate. British Medical Journal 292: 79–80
Riss B, Thomsen K, Christiansen C 1987 Does calcium supplementation prevent postmenopausal bone loss? A double blind controlled clinical study. New England Journal of Medicine 316: 173–177
Wright V (ed) 1983 Bone and joint disease in the elderly. Churchill Livingstone, Edinburgh

21. DISEASES OF THE JOINTS

OSTEOARTHRITIS

Osteoarthritis results from damage to the avascular hyaline cartilage of the synovial joints. Almost any of the synovial joints may be affected. In the lower limbs the knees, hips and metatarsophalangeal joints are most commonly involved and in the upper limbs the elbows and shoulders.

The incidence increases with age and surveys show that almost all individuals over 65 years have X-ray evidence of osteoarthritic changes, but only 15–20% have clinical symptoms.

Clinical features

Knees

— In the early stages the chief symptom is pain during certain activities, e.g. climbing stairs. The stiffness is often worse after a period of immobility. There may be pain on passive flexion and some wasting of the quadriceps

— Later the knee loses its full range of movement. The limitation of extension leads to loss of stability, with the complaint that the knee gives way

— Even later the medial compartment of the knee becomes the most severely affected, producing a genu varum deformity. The patient's balance may be impaired owing to alteration in the centre of balance

— An effusion may occur (more often in the knee than in the other joints). The synovial inflammatory reaction probably develops in response to loose particles of degenerated cartilage within the joint. A synovial cyst may form which can produce a cystic swelling in the popliteal fossa (Baker's cyst)

Hips

The patient walks with a painful limp and has difficulty in managing stairs and in getting in and out of a low chair or a bath. When both hips are affected the patient is much more severely disabled and walks with a shuffling gait.

Upper Limb Joints

Osteoarthritis of the larger joints, shoulder, elbow and wrist, produces stiffness and painful restriction of movement without marked deformity.

Generalized osteoarthritis

— Primary generalized osteoarthritis of Kellgren and Moore (1952) often appears in women at the time of the menopause. The joints most frequently affected are the distal interphalangeal joints of the fingers, the first carpometacarpal joints, the big toes and the first metatarsal joints, the interfacetal joints of the spine, the knees and the hips

— Involvement of the distal interphalangeal joints produces Heberden's nodes and of the proximal interphalangeal joints leads to the less common Bouchard's nodes

— The onset is relatively acute with extreme tenderness of the joints; the skin over the joints may be reddened and warm. The acute phase subsides after a few months. There is no constitutional disturbance, but the erythrocyte sedimentation rate may be moderately raised. This, together with polyarticular involvement, may lead to the mistaken diagnosis of rheumatoid arthritis

Treatment of osteoarthritis

Much can be done to relieve symptoms and to improve function. When the weight-bearing joints are affected in obese patients, dietary restriction is desirable.

Physiotherapy

— Local treatment with radiant heat, short-wave diathermy and wax baths may produce temporary benefit. More worthwhile results are achieved when this kind of treatment is combined with active exercises

— The purpose of active exercises is to break a vicious circle of pain in the joint, muscle inhibition, muscle atrophy, joint instability and worsening of the arthritis. Thus physiotherapy can improve the strength of the muscles, the range of movement of the joint and the function of the joint

Drug therapy

— Simple analgesics, such as aspirin and paracetamol, can be used for the relief of pain. In the elderly high doses of aspirin should be avoided

— Non-steroidal anti-inflammatory drugs (NSAID) are more effective than simple analgesics. They must, however, be used with great caution owing to the danger of gastric erosion and haemorrhage, the frequency of which increases with age. A gastroscopic study has shown that nearly one-quarter of patients receiving a single drug and one-half of those receiving combined treatment with more than one drug had gastric erosions

— NSAIDs which are most often used are listed in Table 21.1. Phenylbutazone and other pyrazoles are poorly tolerated and should not now be prescribed

Table 21.1 Commonly used NSAIDs

Class	Drug	Daily dosage
Indenes	Indomethacin	50–200 mg
	Sulindac	200–400 mg
Proprionic acid derivatives	Ibuprofen	1.2–1.8 g
	Ketoprofen	100–200 mg
	Fenoprofen	0.9–2.4 g
	Flurbiprofen	150–200 mg
	Fenbufen	600–900 mg
	Naproxen	500–1000 mg
Fenamates	Mefanamic acid	1.5 g
	Flufenamic acid	400–600 mg
Aryl acetic acid derivatives	Fenclofenac	600–1200 mg
	Diclofenac	75–150 mg
Oxicams	Piroxicam	20 mg

Intra-articular steroids
— The drugs commonly used are dexamethasone, hydrocortisone, methyl prednisolone and prednisolone. They are more likely to be of benefit when inflammation and synovial effusion (which should be aspirated first) are present
— Repeated injections carry a risk of infection. Degenerative changes in the joint similar to those occurring in Charcot's joints have been reported but are rare

Surgery
The operations of choice now are total joint replacement for the hip and knee. Various types of prostheses are available and with the newer types over 90% of patients benefit, often considerably.

SPONDYLOSIS

— On the basis of X-ray changes spondylosis is almost universal after the age of 70 years, but there is no clear relationship between these changes and symptoms. Clinical manifestations are most often present when spondylosis affects the cervical and lumbar spine
— Spondylosis arises from degeneration of the intervertebral discs and must be distinguished from osteoarthritis of the spine, which affects the apophyseal joints. The two conditions often occur together

Clinical features

Cervical spondylosis
— In a review of 100 cases Brain et al (1952) found that the commonest presenting neurological features were brachial

root pain (32%), headache (28%), giddiness (17%), vertebrobasilar insufficiency (5%), attacks of unconsciousness (4%) and drop attacks (3%)

— Cervical myelopathy due to cord compression is the most serious manifestation. It is characterized by long tract signs in the lower limbs, namely weakness, progressive impairment of the gait and dragging the feet when walking; the paraplegia is rarely severe enough to produce immobility. Mild to moderate ataxia in the legs may be present

— The patient may complain of paraesthesiae and numbness in the fingers, and there may be heaviness and clumsiness of hand movements

— Changes in the tendon reflexes are determined by the level at which major involvement of the cord occurs. When the site is at the C5 intervertebral disc a characteristic finding is reversal of the supinator jerk (inverted radial reflex). Tapping the lower end of the radius produces reflex flexion of the fingers; the biceps jerk may be absent and the triceps reflex exaggerated

— Impairment of function of the mechanoreceptors in cervical spondylosis causes disturbance of balance (see p. 251)

Lumbar spondylosis

— The presenting symptom is usually backache. Radicular pain, for example, in sciatica or in the anterior thigh due to L4 lesions is the result of osteophytic involvement of nerve root foramina

— Pain of sudden onset due to acute intervertebral disc protrusion is common in the elderly. One study has shown that the upper lumbar nerve roots are more often involved in the elderly than in the young, and the predominant feature is pain in the groin or thigh which can be mistaken for disease of the hip

— Some patients with spondylosis also have spondylolisthesis. This is usually at the L4–5 level or the L5–S1 level; it produces backache. The condition is readily diagnosed on X-ray examination

Management

Cervical spondylosis

— The majority of patients who have no symptoms do not require treatment

— Radicular symptoms respond to the use of a collar. The aim is to restrict the normal neck movements, which damage the abnormally fixed cord. Not only are local symptoms relieved, but further damage to the cord may be prevented

— A collar made from Plastizote is more effective and

comfortable than a rigid plastic collar. It should be worn continuously and especially at night, when the symptoms due to nerve root compression tend to be worse. The length of time the collar has to be worn is variable and depends on the response. In favourable cases it can be as short as 2–3 weeks

— The patient with an acute onset of radicular symptoms and evidence of cord compression should be treated promptly by lying him flat in bed and immobilizing the head with sandbags or a collar. A myelogram is indicated after the acute phase has subsided and a neurosurgical opinion should be sought

Lumbar spondylosis
— The majority of cases are asymptomatic and for these patients no treatment is indicated
— There is no especially effective method of management, be it physiotherapy, manipulation, analgesic drugs or a corset
— The pain of an acute lumbar disc protrusion usually subsides after a few days rest in bed. During the acute phase analgesic agents are required. Epidermal steroid injection (methyl prednisolone in normal saline) is often valuable in the relief of severe pain due to nerve root compression

RHEUMATOID ARTHRITIS

Rheumatoid arthritis is a systemic disorder which predominantly affects the smaller peripheral joints through inflammation and proliferative changes in the synovial membrane. Later there is erosion of the articular cartilage and destruction of the supportive structures, with the production of joint deformities.

Prevalence
— Although less common than osteoarthritis rheumatoid arthritis is a crippling disease of long duration and sufficiently prevalent in old age as to constitute an important clinical problem
— In younger patients the disease affects women predominantly but with advancing age the sex differential tends to disappear and after the age of 70 the ratio M:F = 2:3

Clinical features

Articular
— Typically the disease is of gradual onset with joint pain, tenderness, warmth, and swelling due to synovitis,

Limitation of movement and impaired joint function are present during the early active phase
— Another salient characteristic is the stiffness following rest and immobility (the 'gel phenomenon') especially noticeable in the morning on rising
— In some cases the articular symptoms are preceded by a prodromal period of constitutional symptoms and diffuse muscular pain
— There is involvement of the peripheral joints, leading to symmetrical polyarthritis affecting the proximal interphalangeal joints, metacarpophalangeal joints, the small joints of the feet, the wrists, elbows, knees, ankles and shoulders. Involvement of the temporomandibular joints causes pain on mastication
— In the hands the typical deformities are:
  • Ulnar deformities at the metarcarpal phalangeal joints with the extensor tendons sliding off the metacarpal heads to the ulnar side. Later subluxation of the joints occurs
  • Swan neck fingers with hyperextension at the proximal interphalangeal joints
  • In the boutonniere deformity there is flexion at the proximal interphalangeal joint and hyperextension at the distal joint
— In the feet similar deformities occur, with upward displacement of the first phalanx and hallux valgus

Periarticular

— Subcutaneous nodules occur in one-quarter to one-third of cases. The most common location is over the olecranon, but they also occur at other sites of pressure
— Tendosynovitis with tendon sheath effusion is found most commonly in the extensor tendons overlying the wrist and the dorsum of the hand
— Entrapment syndromes occur, e.g. carpal tunnel syndrome, which is due to compression of the median nerve at the wrist. The patient complains of numbness and pain, especially at night, with disturbance of sleep

Vascular

— Raynaud's phenomenon is the most common vascular lesion in rheumatoid disease, occurring in about one-fifth of cases
— In some cases peri-ungual infarcts develop with finger ischaemia which may progress to gangrene
— A characteristic manifestation of vasculitis is ulceration, most commonly over the dorsal surface of the ankle
— Pericarditis occurs in a high proportion of cases but it is rarely symptomatic

Neurological
— Peripheral neuropathy probably results from vasculitis of the vasa nervorum. The sensory form is the most common, with paraesthesiae in the lower limbs. Motor nerve involvement may present as wrist drop, (see p. 174). Recurrent laryngeal nerve paralysis leads to hoarseness
— Vertebral subluxations in the cervical spine, especially at the atlanto-axial and C3–C4 levels, are common in the later stages of the disease. In a small proportion of cases cervical cord compression can result. Acute paraplegia may follow trauma such as a fall from a chair or bed

Pulmonary
— The pulmonary manifestations of rheumatoid disease are more common in men
— Pleural effusions occur especially at times of increased disease activity
— Diffuse interstitial fibrosis (fibrosing alveolitis) may be found, particularly in sero-positive patients
— Nodular lesions are probably vasculitic in origin and are similar to the granulomatous subcutaneous nodes
— Caplan's syndrome is a rheumatoid pneumoconiosis which has been reported in Welsh miners with rheumatoid disease and is attributed to exposure to coal dust

Ocular
— Sjogren's syndrome with xerophthalmia is the most common ocular manifestation
— Scleral and episcleral inflammatory lesions associated with general vasculitis occur less frequently

Different pattern of the disease in the elderly
In the older patient there is:
1. A higher incidence of shoulder joint involvement. The condition may start with pain and stiffness in the shoulder and hand (simulating the shoulder–hand syndrome). Dislocation of the shoulder may occur in the chronic stages and this is often in an upward direction in the patient who uses a walking frame
2. Deformity is usually less and the prognosis more benign in spite of more severe radiological changes
3. The erythrocyte sedimentation rate is often markedly elevated out of proportion to the degree of constitutional disturbance
4. Poor prognosis in the elderly is associated with an insidious onset, strong seropositivity for rheumatoid factor and the presence of extra-articular disease

Diagnosis

The following conditions have to be considered in differential diagnosis
- — Primary generalized osteoarthritis
- — Psoriatic arthritis
- — Polyarticular gout
- — Pyrophosphate arthropathy
- — Malignant arthropathy
- — Polymyalgia rheumatica

Management

General measures
- — Treatment demands a careful balance between rest and activity. Rest is essential in the active phase with constitutional disturbances, but prolonged immobilization, especially with faulty positioning, can lead to serious disability and crippling disablement
- — During the active phase careful attention must be paid to the optimum position of the affected joints. Light PVC or Plastazote splints moulded to the limbs may be required, especially for the wrists and knees. The patient is often tempted to place a pillow behind the knees to gain comfort; this must be resisted since even slight persistent flexion deformity can prevent the patient walking
- — As the active phase of the disease passes, a wide variety of exercises should be carried out. These should be related to activities required for daily living. Such purposeful exercises are valuable means of improving joint function and improving muscle strength. The patient should be reassured that the crippling disablement which was formerly common can now be prevented by the use of newer anti-inflammatory drugs

Drug therapy

Non-steroidal anti-inflammatory drugs (NSAIDs)
- — In using NSAIDs attention must be paid to the total dosage, the time of administration, and the duration of action. Ideally the patient should have a rapidly acting agent in the morning, a second dose in the late afternoon and a long-acting preparation at night in order to ensure sleep and to reduce morning stiffness
- — Information on appropriate NSAIDs for use in the elderly is given on page 195. Long-acting drugs, e.g. naproxen, can be given 12-hourly and have a high therapeutic ratio. In any particular patient the best NSAID cannot always be predicted and it may be necessary to try several agents before the most effective is found

Chrysotherapy
— Gold is often an effective treatment and provided there are no side effects it can be given indefinitely. Sodium aurothiomalàte (myocrysin) should be given intramuscularly in a weekly dose of 10 mg (originally a dose of 50 mg was given but this is no more effective than the smaller dose). In patients who respond a 50 mg monthly maintenance dose can be used
— Gold once absorbed into the body is not excreted. The common toxic effects are renal damage, blood dyscrasias, skin rashes and stomatitis. Hepatitis, colitis and polyneuropathy are less common. Each dose should be monitored by urinalysis and a leucocyte count

D-Penicillamine
— D-Penicillamine has been shown to decrease joint inflammation and the gel phenomenon, and to increase grip strength after 6 months of treatment. It is often reserved for patients who have not responded to NSAID therapy alone. The dose initially is 125–250 mg daily, increasing by the same amount at 4–12-week intervals. Maintenance dose is usually 500–750 mg daily
— Skin rashes and stomatitis are the most common early toxic reactions. More serious adverse reactions are drug fever, renal damage, hepatocellular necrosis, leucopenia, thrombocytopenia and aplastic anaemia. Monitoring by urinalysis and blood counts should be carried out as in the case of gold therapy

Hydroxychloroquine
— Hydroxychloroquine has replaced chloroquine owing to its lower toxicity. Usually it is given in a dose of 200 mg nightly, together with an NSAID. Improvement may be expected in 3–6 months of treatment; if a remission occurs a maintenance dose can be continued indefinitely
— The most serious adverse reaction is retinal damage, which can lead to visual loss. Ophthalmological examination at 6-monthly intervals should be carried out

Corticosteroids
— Corticosteroids given orally should be used with caution in the elderly owing to the high incidence of side effects, notably osteoporotic vertebral collapse in both sexes
— The main indications for steroids are
  • An explosive onset of polyarthritic involvement
  • Severe disease refractory or intolerant of NSAID therapy
  • Vasculitis not controlled by other means
— Intra-articular steroids (dexamethasone sodium phosphate

1–4 mg, hydrocortisone acetate 5–50 mg) are often helpful
during phases of acute or recurrent joint inflammation

Immunosuppressives
Several immunosuppressive agents, e.g. azathioprine, cyclophosphamide
or chlorambucil, can be helpful in refractory cases.

Surgery
The main role of orthopaedic surgery is in total joint replacement,
especially of the hips and knees.

GOUT

The most characteristic manifestation of gout is an intense articular
inflammation due to intracellular sodium urate crystals in the synovial
fluid.

Clinical features
— The peak incidence of acute gout is in males in the fourth
  and fifth decade. Rather more than 10% of patients have
  their first attack after the age of 60 years. The disease is
  rare in premenopausal women
— In later life, the development of gout is often associated
  with blood dyscrasias producing increased cellular activity
  and with the use of thiazide diuretics
— Typically only one joint is affected and in 70% of cases it is
  the metatarsal phalangeal joint of the big toe. The joint
  becomes red, shiny, swollen and intensely tender. Other
  joints which may be involved are those of the foot, fingers,
  the wrist, knees and elbows. Occasionally several joints are
  affected simultaneously — the polyarticular form
— In chronic tophaceous gout deposits of sodium urate occur
  in the periarticular tissues, e.g. in the distal interphalangeal
  joints, causing the skin to become red and shiny and
  sometimes progressing to ulceration. Articular structures
  may be destroyed, with the development of secondary
  degenerative arthritis
— Tophi occur in other sites, particularly the external cartilage
  of the ear, the olecranon and prepatellar bursae, and the
  Achilles tendons

Diagnosis
— The definitive diagnosis can be made by the identification of
  crystals of sodium urate in the synovial fluid. These can
  usually be seen by using ordinary light microscopy, but are
  best detected by means of a polarizing microscope
— Serum uric acid level is raised, but the presence of a high
  level is not always due to gouty arthritis. In differential

diagnosis the conditions listed on page 200 must be
considered

Treatment

Acute attack
— Colchicine was formerly the drug of choice. Although still
  used it commonly produces side effects. Indomethacin and
  phenylbutazone have largely been replaced by the newer
  NSAIDs
— Among the drugs which have been shown to be effective are
  • Naproxen, as a single dose of 750 mg followed by doses
    of 250 mg three times a day
  • Fenoprofen, 1800 mg 6-hourly for 5 days
  • Piroxicam, 40 mg once daily for 5 days
  • Fenbufen, given in divided doses of 600–1000 mg daily

Long-term treatment
— In chronic tophaceous gout with the presence of acute
  attacks of gouty arthritis the serum uric acid level should be
  lowered. Both probenecid and allopurinol are well tolerated,
  although acute attacks can continue during the first few
  months of treatment with either drug
— Allopurinol is to be preferred in patients who have large
  tophaceous deposits, renal failure, urate stones and in gout
  secondary to blood dyscrasias
— There is some evidence that the decline in renal function
  which occurs in untreated patients and those treated with
  colchicine alone does not occur when the colchicine is
  combined with allopurinol

PYROPHOSPHATE ARTHROPATHY (PSEUDOGOUT)

This is a disease of advancing age, and in one series the mean age was
over 70 years. It is due to crystal deposition of calcium pyrophosphate
dihydrate (CPPD).

Clinical features
— In acute gout the big toe is typically affected but in
  pyrophosphate arthropathy it is most commonly the knee
  and other larger joints (hips and shoulders) rather than the
  smaller joints
— The clinical course is variable; some patients have only
  occasional attacks, whereas others develop a progressive
  degenerative joint disease without acute attacks
— Acute attacks can be precipitated by many medical illnesses,
  surgical operations, blood transfusion and by diuretics

Diagnosis

— The diagnosis can be confirmed by the finding of CPPD crystals in synovial fluid. When examined with a polarizing microscope the crystals show weak, positive birefringence

— A characteristic in pyrophosphate arthropathy is the finding on X-ray examination of articular calcification (chondrocalcinosis). This is most commonly seen in the menisci of the knee and in the symphysis pubis. It also occurs in the synovial membrane and capsule around the larger joints e.g. the hip and shoulder

Treatment

— The treatment of an acute attack is similar to that of gout. An acute attack in the knee can often be relieved by joint aspiration; if this alone is ineffective it can be followed by the intra-articular injection of corticosteroids

— The treatment of chronic symptomatic degenerative joint disease associated with pyrophosphate deposition is similar to that of osteoarthritis using a variety of means (see p. 194). Surgical correction of joint deformities with severe pain is often of considerable benefit

MALIGNANT ARTHROPATHY

Hypertrophic pulmonary osteoarthropathy

This is the commonest condition, associated with a variety of intrathoracic tumours, but particularly bronchogenic carcinoma. Although a much rarer condition, pleural mesothelioma frequently leads to hypertrophic osteoarthropathy.

Clinical features

— The salient feature is clubbing of the fingers and toes, and enlargement of the extremities resulting from periarticular and periosteal thickening

— The joints may be swollen, painful and warm. The amount of pain is variable. A painful polyarthropathy resembling rheumatoid disease can occur

— There may be thickening of the skin of the face, leading to coarsening of the features

— X-ray examination shows periosteal thickening and new bone formation. It is often seen at the wrists, but can be found at other sites

Treatment

— Removal of the primary tumour may lead to complete resolution of the arthropathy. Sometimes unilateral or bilateral vagotomy is of benefit

— In the absence of response to these procedures, corticosteroids and antirheumatic drugs should be given

Malignant polyarthritis

A form of arthritis resembling rheumatoid disease has been reported in patients with cancer, notably the lymphomas. There is, however, no conclusive evidence that this is a distinct entity. The onset is often acute; the distribution of joint involvement is asymmetrical, with a tendency to spare the wrist and fingers.

NEUROPATHIC ARTHROPATHY

This form of arthropathy is comparatively rare, but it should be suspected when an elderly patient presents with a gross destructive condition of a joint and with little or no pain.

Clinical features

— When motor function is preserved, but the ability to perceive pain is impaired, the joint is subjected to abnormal stresses without the protective function normally provided by pain. The most common causes are tabes dorsalis (Charcot's joints), syringomyelia, diabetic neuropathy and the repeated intra-articular injection of corticosteroids (see p. 201)

— In tabes the larger joints of the lower limbs are most involved but it may affect the spine and the joints of the upper limb. In syringomyelia the upper limb joints are usually affected and in diabetic neuropathy it is most often the tarsal joints that show degenerative changes. There is typically painless swelling of the foot, without redness and warmth; as the condition progresses the foot becomes shortened and deformed

— In spite of the severe destructive arthropathy the patient continues to use the joint owing to the absence of pain and by the time he seeks medical attention the condition is often advanced

Treatment

When a large weight-bearing joint such as a knee is affected, support by splinting should be used in an attempt to provide extra stability.

CAPSULITIS OF THE SHOULDER

This again is a common condition in the elderly. It may arise spontaneously but more often results from a painful condition which immobilizes the shoulder, such as angina, ischaemic heart disease or hemiplegia.

Clinical features

— The main feature is pain around the shoulder, with limitation of movement, particularly an inability to raise the arm for such activities as dressing and brushing the hair
— When tested with the scapula fixed, examination reveals a loss of passive movements of the shoulder as well as difficulty in raising the arm actively

Treatment

Active treatment with exercises to increase the range of movement is usually practised and is effective. In most cases it must be combined with the use of analgesic drugs and sometimes with the injection of hydrocortisone.

SHOULDER–HAND SYNDROME

This condition occurs when the shoulder is immobilized by hemiplegia and when there is long continued pain in the shoulder due, for example, to capsulitis and ischaemic heart disease.

Clinical features

— There is diffuse tender swelling of the fingers in association with a stiff shoulder. Later the vasomotor changes may lead to atrophy of the skin
— X-ray examination reveals patchy osteoporosis of the head of the humerus and the bones of the wrist and hand

Treatment

It is usual to prescribe active and passive movements of the shoulder and finger joints in order to counteract the atrophy of the skin, the wasting of the muscles and the loss of bone.

BIBLIOGRAPHY

Brain W R, Northfield D, Wilkinson M 1952 The neurological manifestations of cervical spondylosis. Brain 75: 187
Doherty M, Dieppe P 1986 Crystal deposition disease in the elderly. Clinics in Rheumatic Diseases 12: 97–116
Gardiner D L 1983 The nature and causes of osteoarthrosis. British Medical Journal 286: 418–424
Healey L A 1986 Rheumatoid arthritis in the elderly. Clinics in Rheumatic Diseases 12: 173–179
Kellgren J H, Moore R 1952 Primary generalised osteoarthrosis. British Medical Journal 1: 181
Wright V (ed) 1983 Bone and joint disease in the elderly. Churchill Livingstone, Edinburgh

22. ACUTE CONFUSIONAL STATES

Definition

The term 'acute confusional state' refers to an altered state of consciousness which has developed over a short period, i.e. hours to days. Nowadays, quite often the term 'brain failure' is used, indicating that when a person is confused, there is some failure of overall brain function. Other terms used to describe an acute confusional state are acute delirium and acute toxic confusional state. However, the use of the word 'toxic' implies ignorance of the cellular and biochemical causes of acute confusion and therefore this term is now being used less frequently.

Epidemiology

Acute confusional states are common in old age. Although an acute confusional state can occur in both young and old, it is much more common in the old and a lesser stimulus is required to produce confusion in an old person than in a young person.

The Royal College of Physicians' study 'Organic Mental Impairment in the Elderly' (1981) found that a quarter of elderly patients judged mentally normal at the time of admission to hospital showed evidence of an acute confusional state during the first month of hospitalization, while more than a third of demented patients appeared to have super-added acute confusional states at some time during their stay in hospital.

Lipowski (1983) found that 10–15% of patients aged 65 years or over experience an acute confusional state after surgery. There is also some evidence that sleep deprivation, fatigue, sensory deprivation consequent upon hearing or visual disabilities, sensory overstimulation, immobilization, a history of previous psychosis or a family history of psychosis, and polypharmacy increase the chance of an acute confusional state.

The common occurrence of acute confusional states in old age can be related to the greater vulnerability of the ageing brain, and this vulnerability is enhanced in those already suffering from degenerative brain disorders such as dementia and parkinsonism. Acute confusional states represent an unfavourable complication of physical disease in old age, but the prospects for mental recovery and for discharge from hospital are good for those surviving the initial illness.

Aetiology

Acute confusion is a common, non-specific presenting symptom of illness in old age. Especially in patients with serious physical illness more than one causal factor may be present. Although there are well-recognized associations between acute confusional states and many physical conditions, there is little understanding of the mechanism of production of the mental disturbances. Acute confusional states may result from disorders of the brain itself, e.g. transient ischaemic attacks or minor cerebrovascular accidents, but mostly they are secondary to physical illness. In many conditions a likely mechanism of action can be postulated, e.g. cerebral hypoxia due to respiratory failure, failure of cerebral perfusion or severe anaemia; in other conditions there may be various factors playing a role in causing the acute confusional state, e.g. in congestive cardiac failure it is uncertain whether cerebral hypoxia is the principal cause or whether other metabolic factors might be responsible; chest infection may produce an acute confusional state through a number of mechanisms — hypoxia, hypercapnia, fever and bacterial toxins may all play a causal role. The physical conditions most commonly associated with acute confusional states in the elderly are

— Chest infection
— Urinary tract infection
— Congestive cardiac failure and/or left ventricular failure
— Carcinomatosis

A more comprehensive list of conditions which are associated with acute confusional states is shown in Table 22.1.

Table 22.1 Conditions associated with acute confusional states

Infections	Chest infection
	Urinary tract infection
	Viral infection
	Septicaemia
	Meningitis
	Encephalitis
	Subacute bacterial endocarditis
	Myocarditis
Cerebral hypoxia	Respiratory failure
	Congestive cardiac failure or left ventricular failure
	Myocardial infarction
	Change of heart rhythm
	Severe anaemia
Cerebral ischaemia	Transient ischaemic attack
	Cerebrovascular accident
	Embolism
	Diffuse cerebrovascular disease
Organic cerebral lesion	Tumour* primary or secondary
	Subdural haematoma*
	Parkinson's disease
Metabolic/endocrine	Hypoglycaemia
	Diabetic precoma
	Hyponatraemia
	Hypokalaemia/hyperkalaemia
	Hypercalcaemia*

	Uraemia/renal failure
	Liver failure
	Dehydration
	Hypothermia
	Hypopituitarism*
	Myxoedema*
	Thyrotoxicosis*
Nutritional	Vitamin B_{12} deficiency*
	Folic acid deficiency*
	Nicotinic acid deficiency*
	Pyridoxine deficiency*
	Riboflavine deficiency*
	Vitamin C deficiency* (scurvy)
	Thiamine deficiency* (Korsakoff's psychosis, Wernicke's encephalopathy)
Venereal disease	Tertiary syphilis*
Drugs	Polypharmacy
	Drugs associated with memory impairment are shown in Table 22.3
	Drugs associated with acute confusional states are shown in Table 22.4
Drug withdrawal	Alcohol
	Corticosteroids
	Hypnotics, including the benzodiazepines
	Opiates
Normal pressure hydrocephalus	A triad of:
	Intellectual failure
	Urinary incontinence
	Apraxia of gait: a slow, unstable, wide based, fixed-footed gait with poor correction, so falls occur frequently
Other causes	Cranial arteritis (giant cell arteritis)
	Sensory deprivation due to hearing or visual disabilities
	Severe psychological stress (sudden bereavement, sudden unexpected or unwanted move)
	Alcoholism
	Insomnia
	Severe pain
	Recent surgery
	Paralytic ileus
	Faecal impaction
	Urinary retention

*Indicates conditions which can also cause subacute confusional state, i.e. a confusional state taking 4 weeks or over to be recognizable.

Clinical features

The classical features are clouding of consciousness and a fluctuating level of awareness. Defects of short-term memory may be accompanied by impairment of recall from long-term memory and by visual hallucinations and misinterpretations.

According to diagnostic criteria DSM-III-R (1987) for acute confusional state there is a sudden reduction of ability to maintain attention to external stimuli (e.g. questions must be repeated because attention wanders) and to shift attention appropriately to new external stimuli (e.g. the patient perseverates an answer to a previous question). Thinking is disorganized, indicated by rambling, irrelevant or incoherent speech.

In addition, again according to the DSM-III-R description, at least two of the following criteria should also be present

1. Reduced level of consciousness, e.g. difficulty keeping awake during examination
2. Perceptual disturbances: illusions and delusions, misinterpretations, hallucinations
3. Disturbance of sleep–wake cycle, with insomnia or daytime sleepiness
4. Increased or decreased psychomotor activity
5. Disorientation to time, place or person
6. Memory impairment, e.g. inability to learn new material, such as the names of several unrelated objects, after 5 minutes, or to remember recent events, such as history of current episode of illness

DSM-III-R requires for the diagnosis of acute confusional state to be made that there is evidence from the history, physical examination, or laboratory tests of a specific organic factor (or factors) judged to be aetiologically related to the disturbance. If this evidence is absent, an aetiological organic factor can be presumed if the confusion cannot be accounted for by any non-organic mental disorder (e.g. manic episode accounting for agitation and sleep disturbance). This implies that (a certain amount of) treatment is possible.

Incomplete clinical pictures are common in elderly patients. Many do not show clouding of consciousness, and hallucinations are infrequent. The clinical features develop over a short period of time. The patient often has intervals during which he appears to be in possession of his mental faculties. Less severe confusional states may be missed unless orientation and memory are tested as can be done by the use of a mental status questionnaire.

Prodromes
These include
— Anxiety
— Restlessness
— Inability to sleep
— Nightmares
— Agitation
— Increased sensitivity to light and sound

Diagnosis
Recognition of the syndrome is the first step towards an accurate diagnosis. Observation of the patient will give valuable information, e.g. chaotic environment, unkempt appearance, ill-looking. Neurological symptoms such as chorea-like movements, myoclonus, ataxia or tremors may or may not be present.

Table 22.2 Aspects of differential diagnosis between acute confusional state and Alzheimer dementia

Acute confusional state	Alzheimer dementia
Clouding of consciousness	Alert
Short history (days)	Longer history (6 months or more)
Acute onset	Slow insidious onset
Marked variability of degree of cognitive impairment with lucid intervals	Slowly progressive deterioration of cognitive function
Short-term memory impaired	Both short- and long-term memory impaired
Anxiety, agitation, fear	No insight into problems, often good facade
Delusions, hallucinations (mostly visual); visual misinterpretations prominent	Delusions (usually occurring in late stages of Alzheimer dementia)
Disorganized thinking and speech, often of lively content	Difficulty in maintaining conversation; answers not to the point, dysphasia may be present
Rapid physical deterioration, patient often seriously ill	Physical deterioration at a late stage
Evidence from physical examination and/or investigations of underlying pathology	Absence of such evidence supports diagnosis of Alzheimer dementia

It is important to obtain an accurate history from someone who knows the patient well (partner, relatives, neighbours, etc.), especially with regard to onset, duration and behavioural aspects. The main aim is to try to determine whether one is dealing with an acute confusional state or dementia. Table 22.2 shows the most important aspects to be taken into account in the differential diagnosis between acute confusional state and dementia. In an acute confusional state there is a history of acute mental impairment of short duration in a patient with a previously normal mental state; in dementia the history is usually one of mental impairment of longer duration with a gradual deterioration over months or even years, possibly in association with self-neglect, urinary incontinence and faecal incontinence. However, this information may not

Table 22.3 Drugs associated with memory impairment

Anticholinergic drugs
Certain anticonvulsants
Certain antihypertensives
Benzodiazepines
Corticosteroids
Phenothiazines
Psychotropic drugs
Sedatives

Table 22.4 Drugs associated with acute confusional states

Amantidine
Anticholinergic drugs
Anticonvulsants
Antidepressants
Antihistamines
Antihypertensives
Antiparkinsonian drugs
Atropine
Centrally acting analgesics
Corticosteroids
Digoxin
Hypoglycaemics
Isoniazid
Opiates
Sedatives
Tranquillizers

Table 22.5 Royal College of Physicians' Mental Test Score

	Score
Name	0/1
Age	0/1
Time (to nearest hour)	0/1
Time of day	0/1
Name and address for recall in 5 minutes; this should be repeated by the patient to ensure it has been heard correctly:	
Mr John Brown	0/1/2
42 West Street	0/1/2
Gateshead	0/1
Day of week	0/1
Date (correct day of month)	0/1
Month	0/1
Year	0/1
Place:	
Type of place (i.e. hospital)	0/1
Name of hospital	0/1
Name of ward	0/1
Name of town	0/1
Recognition of two persons (doctor, nurse, etc.)	0/1/2
Date of birth (day and month sufficient)	0/1
Place of birth (town)	0/1
School attended	0/1
Former occupation	0/1
Name of wife, sibling or next of kin	0/1
Date of World War I (year sufficient)	0/1
Date of World War II (year sufficient)	0/1
Name of present monarch	0/1
Name of present prime minister	0/1
Months of year backwards	0/1/2
Count 1–20	0/1/2
Count 20–1	0/1/2
Maximum total score	34 points
Score > 28 points	no cognitive impairment
Borderline score	24–28 points

The higher the score the less the degree of cognitive impairment. From Roth M, Hopkins B 1953 Psychological test performance in patients over sixty: 1. Senile psychosis and the affective disorders of old age. Journal of Mental Science 99: 439–450.

Table 22.6 Mini-Mental State Examination

Orientation
Score one point for each correct answer to the following:
1. What is the time? day? date? month? year?	5 points
2. What is the name of this ward? hospital? district? town? country?	5 points

Registration
3. Examiner names three objects. Score up to 3 points if, at the first attempt, the patient repeats, in order, the three objects. Score 2 or 1 if this is the number of objects he repeats correctly. Use further attempts and prompting so that he may be asked to recall them later	3 points

Attention and calculation
4. Ask the patient to subtract 7 from 100, and then 7 from the result. Repeat this 5 times down to 65, scoring 1 point for each correct subtraction	5 points

Recall
5. Ask for the three objects in the registration test, scoring 1 for each	3 points

Language
6. Score 1 point for each of two objects correctly named (pencil and watch).	2 points
7. Score 1 point for correct repetition of this phrase: 'No ifs, ands or buts'	1 point
8. Score 3 if a three-stage command is correctly executed or 1 for each stage. For example, 'with the right index finger touch the tip of your nose and then your left ear'	3 points
9. On a blank piece of paper write 'CLOSE YOUR EYES'. Ask the patient to obey: score 1 point	1 point
10. Ask the patient to write one short sentence with a subject and a verb	1 point

Construction and spatial sense
11. Construct a pair of intersecting pentagons, each side 1 inch long. Score 1 if this is correctly copied	1 point
Maximum total score	30 points

Interpretation of result
— Score 24–30 points: no cognitive impairment; however, memory impairment may be present
— Score 20–23 points: mild cognitive impairment
— Score 14–19 points: moderate cognitive impairment
— Score 0–13 points: severe cognitive impairment

Adapted from Folstein M F, Folstein S E, McHugh P R 1975 Mini-mental state: A practical method for grading the cognitive state of patients for the clinician. Journal of Psychiatric Research 12: 189–198.

be available and a patient may have mild or moderate dementia without the diagnosis ever having been established, especially if it concerns an elderly person living alone.

A full drug history must be obtained; drugs associated with memory impairment are shown in Table 22.3; drugs associated with acute confusional states are shown in Table 22.4; polypharmacy increases the chance of an acute confusional state.

For the detection of organic mental impairment several mental status questionnaires are available, which test for short- and long-term memory, orientation, awareness of events, and ability to count forwards and backwards. They are a convenient and reliable method of assessment.

Commonly used questionnaires are The Royal College of Physicians Mental Status Questionnaire (Table 22.5), Hodkinson's Abbreviated Mental Test Score, and Folstein's Mini-Mental State Examination (Table 22.6). The patient's educational level must be taken into account. Depression, dysphasia, deafness, visual impairment, drug intoxication, physical illness and a change in environment can all reduce the score. The mental state examination is incomplete unless orientation and memory have been checked and recorded. The numerical score obtained by the patient during the acute confusional spell should serve only as a baseline value and should never be considered a status quo, e.g. after treatment of the underlying pathology the mental status questionnaire should be repeated and ought to show improvement; one might find that an abnormal score has turned into a normal or near-normal one. It is best to avoid the first 24 hours after admission for obtaining a mental test score because the patient is in unfamiliar surroundings and will need time to settle first. Take your time and explain to the patient that you will ask him some questions (try to avoid the word 'test').

Korsakoff's psychosis
There is a strong history of alcohol ingestion; the most remarkable clinical feature is loss of short-term memory and confabulation in the absence of other evidence of dementia.

Investigations
An acute confusional state in an elderly person should be considered a medical emergency. Whether the patient's mental state improves depends greatly on the physician's approach and the treatment of any underlying pathology.

Physical examination
- — Neurological examination (check for evidence of dysphasia and parietal lobe signs)
- — Fundoscopy
- — Measuring rectal temperature, if necessary with a low-reading rectal thermometer
- — Check for faecal impaction (including rectal examination)
- — Check for urinary retention

Laboratory investigations
- — ESR
- — Full blood count (FBC)
- — Urea and electrolytes

— Serum creatinine level
— Serum glucose level
— Serum calcium level
— Liver function tests
— Thyroid function tests
— Serum vitamin B_{12} level $\Big\}$ (on indication, i.e.
— Serum folate level $\quad\Big|$ if MCV is raised)
— Blood cultures (on indication, i.e. slightly raised temperature plus the presence of a cardiac murmur could indicate subacute bacterial endocarditis)
— Cardiac enzymes (on indication, i.e. confusion of very recent onset could be due to a 'silent myocardial infarction')
— Determination of drug levels (on indication, i.e. serum digoxin level)
— Microscopic analysis and culture of urine

Technical investigations
— Chest X-ray
— Abdominal film (on indication, i.e. abdominal signs, suspicion of faecal loading)
— ECG
— 24-hour electrocardiographic monitoring (on indication)
— Echocardiography (on indication)

Neurological investigations
— Lumbar puncture
— Skull X-ray
— EEG
— CT scan of the brain

They should be applied when there are specific clinical indications, i.e. if lesions such as cerebral tumour, subdural haematoma or normal pressure hydrocephalus are suspected.

EEG has potential value in distinguishing acute confusional state from dementia.

Management
Treatment of underlying pathology should commence as soon as possible since prompt treatment can reverse the acute confusional state.

General measures
— Reassuring and reorientating the patient constantly
— Maintaining a calm environment; a quiet, well-lit room with one or two familiar objects (such as a well-loved photograph), physical comfort and an unchanging routine all help to reduce alarm
— Restoring and/or maintaining hydration, as dehydration may lead to further deterioration of the patient's physical and mental state
— Recording urine output (fluid balance, urinary retention)
— Recording bowel movements (faecal impaction)

Once the most accurate diagnosis has been reached symptomatic control
of behaviour can be achieved by prescribing medication to control
overactivity or other florid features; these drugs need to be used in the
lowest possible dose and only have a place when the patient is so
restless that he is getting exhausted.

Preparations include the major and minor tranquillizers and
chlormethiazole, which does not belong to either group but has a useful
place in the management of an acute confusional state.

Major tranquillizers
There are two groups in common use
1. Phenothiazines: chlorpromazine, promazine, thioridazine,
   trifluoperazine, fluphenazine
   — Contraindications
     Absolute
     • Sensitivity to phenothiazines
     Relative
     • Bone marrow depression
     • Liver failure
     • Renal failure
     • Severe cardiovascular disease
     • Epilepsy
     • Parkinsonism
   — Side effects
     • Drowsiness, fatigue
     • Skin rash
     • Benign obstructive jaundice
     • (Orthostatic) hypotension
     • ECG changes
     • Epileptiform seizures
     • Parkinsonism
     • Acute dystonias (spasms of eye, face, neck and back
       muscles)
     • Tardive dyskinesia
     • Hypothermia
     • Blurring of vision ⎤
     • Dry mouth   ⎟ anticholinergic side
     • Constipation   ⎟ effects
     • Urinary retention ⎦
     • Bone marrow depression (rare)
   — Most commonly used drugs
     • Chlorpromazine
       – Start with 25 mg od or bd orally, increasing
         gradually if necessary to 25–50 mg tds or qds
       – A preparation for intramuscular injection is
         available, 25–50 mg, to be administered as a single

        dose or repeated at 6–8 hourly intervals, if
necessary
- Has long duration of action and strong side effects
- Promazine
    - 25–50 mg od to tds orally
    - Has fewer side effects than chlorpromazine
- Thioridazine
    - 10–50 mg od to tds orally

2. Butyrophenones: haloperidol
    — Contraindications
    Relative
    - Severe cardiovascular disease
    - Epilepsy
    - Parkinsonism
    — Side effects
    - As for phenothiazines
    — Usual dose
    - 0.5–1 mg bd or tds orally, increasing gradually if necessary to a maximum of 5 mg bd or tds orally
    - When control is achieved reduce to lowest possible dose
    - A preparation for intramuscular injection 5 mg/ml is available

Minor tranquillizers
1. Barbiturates: phenobarbitone, sodium amytal
    — They have been used for many years but nowadays the benzodiazepines are prescribed far more often, because barbiturates are addictive and cause microsomal induction which can upset the dosage of other drugs; in addition, they are themselves a cause of confusion in the elderly
2. Benzodiazepines: chlordiazepoxide, diazepam, oxazepam, lorazepam, temazepam
    — Contraindications
    Absolute
    - Sensitivity to benzodiazepines
    - Myasthenia gravis
    — Side effects
    Unusual and not serious
    - Sleepiness, 'hangover effect'
    - Drowsiness
    - Skin rash
    - Muscular spasm (very rare)
Note:
— Repeated doses may lead to accumulation of drug metabolites
— It has been found that in the elderly plasma

concentration of the intermediate-acting benzodiazepine
temazepam increases by 50% after 7 days of use
— Dose should be kept to a minimum
— Withdrawal should be gradual because of the risk of a
rebound syndrome

Most commonly used benzodiazepines for daytime sedation
— Chlordiazepoxide: a long-acting benzodiazepine
  • Usual dose: 5–20 mg tds orally
— Diazepam: a long-acting benzodiazepine
  • Usual dose: 2–10 mg tds orally
  • A preparation for intramuscular injection of 10 mg is
    available
— Oxazepam: an intermediate-acting benzodiazepine
  • start with 10 mg daily orally; increasing gradually if
    necessary to 10–20 mg tds or qds

Most commonly used benzodiazepine for night-time sedation
— Temazepam: an intermediate-acting benzodiazepine
  • Start with 5 mg at night orally
  • Maximum dose is 20 mg at night orally

Chlormethiazole

This drug has a molecular structure similar to vitamin B_1 or thiamine; it
is now thought to be an 'intermediate' tranquillizer, having a potency
half way between the minor and major tranquillizers. The plasma
half-life is short, about 4 hours; it has a place in the management of
acute confusional states and is used when chlorpromazine or haloperidol
is not producing the desired effect; it should not be given concurrently
with these drugs because of the risk of potentiation of effect.
— Contraindications
  Absolute
  • Acute respiratory failure
  Relative
  • Chronic pulmonary disease
  • Chronic liver disease
  • Chronic renal disease
— Side effects (rare)
  • Sedation, excitement, confusion
  • Conjunctival irritation
  • Nasal congestion
  • Gastrointestinal disturbances
  • Anaphylactic reactions
— Usual dose
  • 1 capsule chlormethiazole 192 mg in Miglyol at night
    orally, with a maximum dose of 2 capsules at night orally
  • 5 ml chlormethiazole edisylate syrup (250 mg/5 ml) at
    night orally, with a maximum dose of 10 ml at night
    orally

Note: 5 ml chlormethiazole edisylate syrup is the equivalent of 1
capsule chlormethiazole 192 mg in Miglyol.

BIBLIOGRAPHY

American Psychiatric Association 1987 Diagnostic and statistical manual of mental disorders, 3rd ed (revised). APA, Washington, DC

Folstein M F, Folstein S E, McHugh P R 1975 Mini-mental state: A practical method for grading the cognitive state of patients for the clinician. Journal of Psychiatric Research 12: 189–198

Hodkinson H M 1972 Evaluation of a mental test score for assessment of mental impairment. Age and Ageing 1: 233–245

Hodkinson H M 1973 Mental impairment in the elderly. Journal of the Royal College of Physicians of London 7: 305

Lipowski Z J 1983 Transient cognitive disorders (delirium, acute confusional states) in the elderly. American Journal of Psychiatry 140: 1426–1436

Report of the Royal College of Physicians on Organic Mental Impairment in the Elderly 1981. Journal of the Royal College of Physicians of London 15: 4–29

Roth M, Hopkins B 1953 Psychological test performance in patients over sixty: 1. Senile psychosis and the affective disorders of old age. Journal of Mental Science 99: 439–450

Solomon S, Hotchkiss E, Saravay S M, Bayer C, Ramsey P, Blum R S 1983 Impairment of memory function by antihypertensive medication. Archives of General Psychiatry 40: 1109–1112

Wood R A 1984 Clinical algorithms: Memory loss. British Medical Journal 288: 1443–1447

23. IMPAIRED VISUAL ACUITY

Age-related changes in the eye

— A gradual hardening of the lens, making it less and less responsive to the ciliary muscle
  - Occurs between the ages of 40 and 65
  - Results in difficulty with reading small print and other forms of near work
    — In previously normal eyes glasses become necessary
    — In previously hypermetropic eyes glasses need to be strengthened
    — In previously myopic eyes glasses may have to be discarded for near work
  - The process is gradual, usually complete by the age of 65
— The lens tends to become larger and opaque; everyone develops some form of opacity in the lens by the time they reach great age. This may result in cataracts
— Pupillary changes
  - There is a decrease in the diameter of the pupil, which reduces the amount of light reaching the retina; this means that for a given task more illumination is required; this is expressed by the patient as 'failing vision by the end of the day'
  - The pupil also responds more slowly to both light and accommodation. This has implications for the lighting of hallways, stairs and passages in the home

In the elderly, significant changes in vision are much more likely to be due to pathological or degenerative processes than in the younger age groups.

MACULAR DEGENERATION

Responsible for about 45% of ocular pathology in the elderly; the macula degenerates owing to impairment of blood supply; in most cases, no specific underlying pathology can be identified and the condition is labelled 'senile macular degeneration'; it is usually bilateral, though the degree of involvement of each eye may differ.

Symptoms
- The macula is responsible for the sharp central vision, when it degenerates a central scotoma develops
- Peripheral vision is retained
- Patient is unable to see small objects clearly and often cannot read or sew

Diagnosis

History
Patient is unable to see small objects clearly; often unable to read or sew or recognize faces; peripheral vision is retained.

Ophthalmoscopy
- In disciform macular degeneration, a subretinal neovascular membrane appears as a well-defined elevated greyish area, often associated with blotchy hyperpigmentation and always with drusen (i.e. small round yellowish lesions deep to the retinal vessels). In the later stages, subretinal haemorrhage may become apparent and finally this is replaced by a white scar
- In the 'dry form' of macular degeneration areas of hypopigmentation occur in the macular region

Treatment
- Only disciform macular degeneration is amenable to specific treatment. Controlled trials have shown that destruction of the subretinal neovascular membrane by laser photocoagulation is beneficial, with useful central vision lasting significantly longer in the treated than in the untreated group, the benefit lasting several years. Careful selection of patients is necessary: the new blood vessels must be away from the fovea and central vision should still be better than 6/36. Laser treatment is more likely to succeed at the early stages. The second eye may be spared for some time, but the patient must be told to return promptly if he notices any distortion of vision in the second eye
- No specific treatment is available for the 'dry form' of macular degeneration
- Aids to maximize the use of existing peripheral vision should be tried; appropriate spectacle correction and good illumination may improve reading; hand magnifiers or a telescope may be helpful
- Reassure the patient that although he may become eligible for registration as partially sighted or blind, he is unlikely to become completely blind

CATARACTS

Cataracts affect about 95% of the population over the age of 65 years to some degree, and account for about 33% of ocular pathology in the elderly; the age of onset varies widely from individual to individual; the development of cataracts is influenced by hereditary tendencies; progression is intermittent and not symmetrical between eyes.

Visual impairment develops if the opacity is situated in or near the centre of the lens or if it is large enough to interfere with the efficient transmission of light.

There is no known method to prevent the formation of cataracts or influence their rate of development.

Symptoms
— Painless, progressive diminution in vision with glare, light sensitivity and multiple images
— Glaucoma may occur as a complication of cataract
   • When the entire lens is affected the degenerated protein may cause the lens to swell; if this swelling is extensive it may displace the iris anteriorly, narrow the anterior chamber angle, and precipitate glaucoma (closed angle type)
   • If the degenerating lens protein becomes liquefied and escapes through the cortex of the lens into the anterior chamber, a lens-protein–macrophage complex may obstruct the chamber angle, interfere with the outflow of aqueous fluid from the anterior chamber and cause glaucoma (phacolytic glaucoma)
   • Urgent specialist advice should be sought if a patient is seen with an advanced cataract and signs of glaucoma
— Occasionally halos around lights may occur owing to deflection of the light by the lens opacity; however, halos around lights are most often due to glaucoma

Diagnosis

History
— Impaired visual acuity which is worse during the day as the pupils constrict
— Check on the use of medication
   • Chronic use of systemic corticosteroids (i.e. more than 10 mg prednisone daily for one year) may cause posterior subcapsular cataract
   • Chlorpromazine may cause anterior capsular and subcapsular lens opacities when used in chronic high doses (i.e. 500 mg daily for 3 years or more); the opacities are golden brown and the visual effect is often mild

- Exposure to radiation (infrared, ultraviolet, X-rays) is another potential cause of cataract

Examination

In senile cataract there are opacities, usually nuclear, with a brownish discoloration, or of the cortical spoke variety.

Management

The treatment of cataracts is surgical excision of the lens, which can now be done without having to wait for the cataract to mature.

Postoperatively the optical problem of the aphakic eye may be solved by employing one of the following

1. A lens implant
2. Various types of contact lenses
3. Traditional spectacles
   — Both (1) and (2) provide the retina with normal-sized visual images; self-insertion of contact lenses is difficult for many elderly patients and their loss is a particular hazard in view of unaided vision being so poor
   — (3) Produces a magnified image, which affects mobility and judgement of distances; sedentary vision remains excellent
   — All three require additional glasses for near vision

GLAUCOMA

Glaucoma accounts for 5% of ocular pathology in the elderly. Glaucoma is found in about 1% of all Europeans over the age of 40, and prevalence increases to 2% at 55 years of age, and to about 10% at 70 years of age.

— Chronic simple glaucoma is the most common type of glaucoma, accounting for about half of all cases

— Incidence increases from about 5/1000 per year at 50 years of age to 10/1000 per year at 70 years of age. The prevalence is increased tenfold when there is a family history of chronic simple glaucoma

— Primary closed angle and congenital glaucoma are each responsible for 10% of cases, with the secondary glaucomas being responsible for the remaining 30% of cases

— There is an increase in intraocular pressure of sufficient magnitude to impair vision: the increased intraocular pressure causes atrophy of the optic disc, with cupping and visual loss

— Ocular hypertension is defined statistically as being above 21 mmHg. The pressure at which glaucomatous optic disc cupping will occur, however, appears to vary between individuals. There is a diurnal variation in intraocular pressure, so repeated measurements over a 24-hour period may be necessary. In some patients the intraocular pressure may be raised only in the supine position

Prevention

— In theory glaucoma is a preventable disease. Reversal of the loss of field and of acuity is not possible after they have been present a relatively short time
— Prevention must be aimed at identifying susceptible eyes and early stages of the disease. Any elderly person whose parents, grandparents or other close relatives suffered from glaucoma should have tonometry every 2 years, and should seek immediate investigation if early symptoms, i.e. episodes of blurred vision or halos around lights, occur
— The earlier treatment is given the more vision will be preserved
— Systemic drugs which may precipitate or aggravate glaucomatous episodes include: mydriatics; drugs with anticholinergic properties; drugs with an atropine-like action; steroids

Closed-angle glaucoma

May present as an acute condition when the angle of the anterior chamber suddenly becomes obstructed and the intraocular pressure rises rapidly; it is usually accompanied by severe headaches (often unilateral), nausea and vomiting. Gastrointestinal symptoms may be so prominent that they can mask the ocular source, which dangerously delays specific treatment.

Diagnosis

— The patient complains of pain in and around the eye, impaired vision, and halos around lights; blurring of vision and visual field defects may occur
— Although the condition is usually bilateral, one eye is frequently more severely affected and appears redder than the other. There is a dilated pupil with a reduced response to light, ciliary injection and a cloudy cornea
— Tonometry reveals a raised intraocular pressure
— Examination of the fundi shows the characteristic cupped appearance of the optic disc
— Gonioscopy indicates a narrow anterior chamber angle

Treatment

— Immediate treatment is sight-saving and consists of instillation of a drop of 2–4% pilocarpine every minute for 5 minutes, followed by a drop every 5 minutes for a half-hour, and then each quarter-hour, until relief or help is obtained. Concurrently acetazolamide should be given: 500 mg orally or 250 mg IV

— Signs of control of the situation
- A reduction in the size of the pupil
- A brighter cornea
- Relief from pain
— Emergency surgery is frequently necessary and consists of surgical or laser iridotomy

Open-angle glaucoma

A chronic, slowly progressive condition, commonest in the elderly; visual loss is peripheral and asymmetric between the eyes, and 6 months to 3 years may pass before significant disability is noticed. The slow rise in intraocular pressure is painless. Patients experience night blindness and loss of mobility vision; without treatment there will be loss of most of the peripheral visual field, sparing central vision until very late and eventually progressing to blindness.

Diagnosis

Signs of optic nerve cupping and loss of peripheral vision are the most important diagnostic features. In earlier stages the diagnosis may be reached by finding an elevated intraocular pressure in the presence of a normal angle. The disease should be suspected in anyone with pale or cupped optic discs.

Treatment

— Treatment consists of controlling intraocular pressure with miotics (e.g. pilocarpine eye drops 0.5–4.0% solution, every 6 hours) and sympathomimetics (e.g. adrenaline eye drops 0.5–1.0% solution tds) which improve aqueous outflow, or with timolol eye drops 0.25 or 0.5% solution tds, which decreases aqueous production
— Oral acetazolamide, 250 mg three or four times daily, may be used for short periods for aqueous inhibition
— Filtration or laser surgery is indicated when there is poor compliance with medical treatment, and when regular monitoring of visual field, optic disc appearance and intraocular pressure demonstrate loss of control
— Life-long follow-up is required
— In secondary glaucoma the cause of ocular hypertension is usually ocular disease

RETINOPATHIES

A number of systemic diseases can interfere with the blood supply of the retina and macula and cause retinal and macular degeneration. These include
— Diabetes mellitus
— Hypertension

— Periarteritis nodosa
— Nephropathies

Diabetic retinopathy

— Particularly common among the elderly diabetic population
— Severity and control of the diabetes do not correlate with the severity of the retinopathy
— In type II diabetes the retinopathy may be present for many years before it is discovered; indeed, the patient may have had a subclinical form of diabetes for many years; these patients ought to be seen by an ophthalmologist within several weeks after discovery of diabetes
— In diabetic hypertensives control of hypertension has been found to be the most important factor in improving the retinopathy
— Treatment of diabetic retinopathy is not satisfactory. Laser photocoagulation may be useful, particularly in early cases (see Ch. 16)

Hypertensive retinopathy

Retinal changes in elderly hypertensive patients usually combine mild abnormalities of both atherosclerotic and hypertensive origin. In younger hypertensive patients narrowing of arterioles is commonly seen; in older people the narrowing is segmental. The earliest change in calibre is reversible, although it is due to arterial thickening with medial hypertrophy. Other segments are dilated with associated medial atrophy. The thickened walls give a heightened light reflex appearing more like copper or silver wire. Veins may show nipping at points of arterial crossing. These early changes may be seen in normotensive individuals with arteriosclerosis. With increasing severity of hypertension retinal haemorrhages and exudates occur. The haemorrhages lying in the nerve-fibre layer are flame-shaped and often lie close to the disc. Soft exudates appear as a greyish area, and rapidly develop into a cotton-wool spot, frequently half as big as the disc itself. They are due to areas of capillary closure with retinal microinfarction. The cotton-wool spot fades and fragments over a period of about 6 weeks. They often spare the macula. Waxy hard-looking exudates are more common in the macula region, with the fovea as the centre of a star of exudates; they may persist.

— Disc oedema occurs in the most severe form of hypertensive retinopathy; the disc is reddened, swollen, and crossed by dilated capillaries
— In the elderly, severe hypertensive retinopathy is rare and suggests a renal or renovascular origin

RETINAL ARTERY OCCLUSION

Occlusion of the retinal artery or one of its branches results in a sudden loss of vision; the extent of the loss of vision depends on the site of the occlusion

1. Occlusion of the central retinal artery results in complete loss of vision in the affected eye
2. Occlusion of one of its branches results in more limited visual loss in the affected eye
   — Sometimes the loss of vision is preceded by amaurosis fugax
   — Direct light pupillary reaction is lost, the consensual reflex is preserved
   — On retinal examination the arteries distal to the occlusion may not be visible or may be replaced by white lines; occasionally the embolus may be seen

Cause
Often due to emboli, for example from an atheromatous plaque in the carotid territory, or from a cardiac source.

Treatment
Emergency treatment must take place within a few minutes to hours and consists of dilatation of the cerebral and retinal arteries, for which various methods have been tried (i.e. increasing arterial carbon dioxide concentration; ocular massage; retrobulbar injection of papaverine; ocular paracentesis). In general, the prognosis of retinal artery occlusion is poor.

RETINAL VEIN OCCLUSION

Occlusion of the retinal vein is often associated with arteriosclerosis and compression of the vein by the sclerotic wall of the adjacent artery and the lamina cribrosa.

— Loss of vision is not as sudden as in retinal artery occlusion and in most cases vision is not completely lost
— Fundoscopy reveals a haemorrhagic retina with markedly congested veins, transudates and oedema
— Treatment with anticoagulants and/or low molecular weight dextran could be tried; however, in many cases cystoid macular oedema develops and the prognosis is poor
— Predisposing systemic diseases are hypertension, diabetes and conditions that slow venous blood flow (hyperviscosity). One-third of these patients have glaucoma

Late complications of the occlusion of a retinal artery or vein include neovascularization glaucoma; the success rate of treatment of this type of glaucoma is very low

Other less frequent ocular causes of impaired vision

— Primary optic atrophy: in cases of disseminated sclerosis and syphilis
— Secondary optic atrophy: secondary to chronic papilloedema
— Optic neuritis: due to demyelinating disorders (rare in old age)
— Retinal tears, retinal detachment
— Haemorrhages in the vitreous humour

Extraocular causes of visual impairment

— Cerebral lesions (see Fig. 23.1)

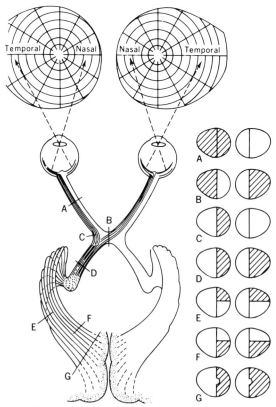

Fig. 23.1 Neurological lesions causing visual field defects. A, Complete blindness in left eye; B, Bitemporal hemianopia; C, Nasal hemianopia of left eye; D, Right homonymous hemianopia; E, F, Right upper and lower quadrant hemianopias; G, Right homonymous hemianopia with preservation of central vision.
From Victor and Adams 1974.

— Giant cell arteritis (see Ch. 19)
— Severe sudden anaemia: may impair the nutrition of the retina and cause blindness (i.e. due to sudden loss of a substantial amount of blood)

Entropion

When most of the lashes are misdirected as a result of permanent inturning of the lid margin (produced classically by the scarring process of trachoma) surgical correction is usually the best method of obtaining permanent relief. In acute involutional entropion (senile entropion) strapping down of the skin of the lower lid will give temporary relief until surgery can be performed.

Ectropion

Usually due to age changes but can also be caused by contracting scar tissue in the skin of the eyelid. This results in a watery eye, because the punctum is held away from the globe. Mild ectropion may be relieved by cautery applied to the tarsal plate, while more severe cases require surgical correction.

Herpes ophthalmicus

Herpes zoster (shingles) is caused by the same virus as chickenpox and may be acquired by chickenpox contacts. The process is confined to the distribution of the first branch (ophthalmic nerve) of the fifth nerve (trigeminal nerve). It is often misdiagnosed in its early stages and mismanaged in its later stages.

Symptoms

— Initial numbness and tingling around the eye, followed in hours or days by redness and swelling of the eyelids
— This swelling often prevents the opening of the lids, and the examiner might have great difficulty in separating them (the swelling may be mistaken for an allergy)
— Pain and tenderness are usually severe
— A spread of oedema across the nose to the other eye may occur; this is merely a spread of oedema, not of the disease
— Swelling and congestion of the conjunctiva is a common early complication
— The oedema begins to resolve after a few days and the eye begins to open
— The formation of skin vesicles may be early and gross or late and minimal
— When the tip of the nose is free from vesicles it is likely that the eye is free from symptoms
— A quiet intraocular inflammation may begin on day 10–14, with a mild decrease in visual acuity

— The safest course is for all patients with shingles to have an ophthalmological opinion within a month of the first symptoms of decrease in visual acuity
— The cornea often becomes anaesthetic; keratitis is then a possibility; if anaesthesia is present an ophthalmologist's opinion is needed within days

Treatment
— Systemic analgesics
— Treatment of the conjunctiva with an antibiotic ointment to prevent secondary infection
— Antiviral agents, e.g. acyclovir, may be given as eye ointment or systemically

Complications
Many patients develop an intractable and often untreatable neuralgia.

EXAMINATION OF THE EYE

— Estimate visual acuity for near and distance *with* glasses
— Small newspaper print will suffice to check reading vision
— Check central fields with an Amsler chart
— Check peripheral fields with the reaction to finger movements between doctor and patient at varying distances from central fixation
— Examine media and retina with ophthalmoscope
— The pinhole test helps in deciding whether different glasses are needed: if an object is viewed through a pinhole almost all refraction is eliminated. Thus, if a patient with defective vision looks at the test card through a pinhole and achieves 6/9 vision, the decreased vision is caused by a refractive error. If the pinhole does not improve visual acuity, organic disease must be suspected
— Measuring intraocular pressure requires training and experience

OPHTHALMOLOGICAL EMERGENCIES

— Sudden loss of vision in one or both eyes (see Table 23.1)
— Giant cell arteritis can cause blindness in both eyes rapidly and irreversibly, whereas central retinal occlusion usually affects one eye

Table 23.1 Causes and features of sudden loss of vision

Site	Cause	Features
Vitreous	Massive vitreous haemorrhage	Loss of red reflex on fundus examination
Retina	Retinal arterial occlusion	Branch: partial loss of vision Central: total loss of vision and of direct pupillary reaction
	Central retinal vein occlusion	Extensive haemorrhage in fundus
	Amaurosis fugax	'Curtain' over vision, usually recovering in minutes Embolus may be visible in retinal arteriole
Optic nerve	Ischaemic optic neuropathy	a. Arteriosclerotic: usually partial visual loss and disc swelling b. Giant cell arteritis: disc swelling. ESR/viscosity raised
	Retinal detachment involving macula	History of flashing lights and peripheral loss extending to central field
	Toxic amblyopia	Quinine or methyl alcohol poisoning
Visual pathway	Stroke	Homonymous hemianopia (the patient may think it unilateral). Total visual loss if previous hemianopia unrecognized or cortical blindness. Normal pupil reactions
	Migraine	Characteristic aura and recovery. Scintillating scotoma; flashing lights. Gastrointestinal symptoms. Recovery almost invariable
Acute glaucoma		Pain ± vomiting Red eye Corneal oedema Semi-dilated pupil Eye stony hard

NB: Apparently sudden visual loss may be due to the discovery of a pre-existing defect or to hysteria. Referral is always justified.
Adapted from Jackson & Finlay (1985).

Laboratory investigations
— ESR
— FBC
— Urea
— Serum creatinine level
— Serum glucose level
— CT scan (on indication)

Low-vision aids
— Optical magnifiers: for near work; all restrict field of vision, rapid scanning becomes impossible

— Telescopes: for distant vision, but field restriction is extreme
— Monocular aids: for identification of bus numbers, street names, etc.
— Closed-circuit television
— Lighting is essential: the elderly eye, whether normal or not, requires more illumination for all visual acts than the young one. Cullinan et al (1979) reported that improvement in domestic lighting would reduce the number of 'visually disabled' at home by nearly 50%.

Registration

A person is eligible for registration as 'blind' when the corrected visual acuity is 3/60 or less, or as 'partially sighted' when it approaches 6/60. Those registered may be given various forms of financial help, including increased rent and rate rebates and half-price rail travel. Those registered as blind may also receive increased supplementary benefit, a high tax allowance, and some television licence rebate. Some local authorities offer the visually handicapped free amenities such as free entry to concerts and free public transport. The Talking Book Service is much appreciated by those unable to read and is available to those registered blind, and to the partially sighted if near vision is poor.

Mobility officers for the blind and partially sighted can give mobility training, and will provide a white stick to warn other people of the visual handicap. A wide range of aids available for the home include large-numeral dials for telephones and Braille knobs for cookers.

— Details are available from the Royal National Institute for the Blind, Public Relations Department, 224 Great Portland Street, London WIN 6AA

BIBLIOGRAPHY

Crick R P 1982 Early detection of glaucoma. British Medical Journal 285: 1063–1064
Cullinan T, Gould E S, Irvine D, Silver J H 1979 Visual disability and home lighting. Lancet 1: 642–644
Gardiner P A 1979 ABC of ophthalmology. British Medical Association, London
Gordon D M 1974 Eye problems of the aged. In: Chuin A B (ed) Working with older people, vol IV: Clinical aspects of ageing. US Department of Health, Education and Welfare, Washington, DC
Hilbourne J F 1975 Social and other aspects of adjustment to cataract extraction in the elderly. Transactions of the Ophthalmological Society of the United Kingdom 95: 254–258
Jackson C R S, Finlay R D (eds) 1985 The eye in general practice, 8th edn. Churchill Livingstone, Edinburgh, Ch 1, p 13
Jones B R 1985 Social responsibilities in ophthalmology. Journal of the Royal Society of Medicine 78: 358–366
Kiljakovic M, Howie J G R, Phillips C I, Bartholomew R S, Brown J G S 1985 Raised intraocular pressure: An alternative method of referral. British Medical Journal 290: 1043–1044
Macular Photocoagulation Study Group 1982 Argon laser photocoagulation for senile macular degeneration: Results of a randomised clinical trial. Archives of Ophthalmology 100: 912–918
Moorfields Macular Study Group 1982 Treatment of senile disciform macular degeneration: a single-blind randomised trial by argon laser photocoagulation. British Journal of Ophthalmology 66: 745–753

Smith R 1984 Laser surgery for glaucoma. Journal of the Royal Society of Medicine 77: 175–177

Steinmann W C 1982 The 'who' and 'how' of detecting glaucoma. British Medical Journal 285: 1091–1093

Victor M, Adams R D 1974 Common disturbances of vision, ocular movement and hearing. In: Wintrobe M M, Isselbacher K J, Petersdorf R G (eds) Harrison's principles of internal medicine, 7th edn. McGraw-Hill Book Company, New York. Ch. 20. p 103

24. DISORDERS OF THE EAR

HEARING IMPAIRMENT

Hearing impairment is common in the elderly and may be apparent on formal testing even in those subjects in the later years of life who deny any hearing impairment. A study of the hearing in 169 subjects in geriatric wards and nursing homes for the elderly showed that every single person, over the age of 60 years, had a significant degree of loss. It is therefore important for the physician to have a clear concept of the diagnosis and management of the various forms of hearing impairment in the elderly patient.

History

Mode of onset
In the elderly the hearing loss is usually of gradual onset, bilateral and symmetrical. Sudden onset, particularly in one ear, may be related to viral infection, barotrauma or head injury. Fluctuating hearing loss may be due to fluid in the middle ear, or Ménière's disease. The past history of the patient may give an indication as to the cause of the hearing loss. Enquiry should be made for past noise exposure, whether in military or civilian occupation, past medication with potentially ototoxic drugs, or of general medical illnesses which can cause damage to the hearing organ such as meningitis and syphilis.

Tinnitus
Hearing loss in the elderly is often accompanied by buzzing noises in the ear. The noises may be high- or low-pitched and continuous or intermittent. They are frequently louder at night when surroundings are quiet. Objective tinnitus may be heard by the clinician on auscultation.

Vertigo
The feeling of unsteadiness may be swaying or rotational. Acute rotational vertigo implies an end-organ lesion.

Ear discharge
This may be due to infection in the external ear canal or middle ear infection discharging through a tympanic membrane perforation.

Earache
This may be due to a local cause in the ear or may be referred from the neck, sinuses or jaw.

Examination of the ear

The pinna and postaural area should be inspected for inflammation, deformity or evidence of previous operation such as depression over the mastoid or a postaural scar. Endaural incisions may be seen anteriorly between the tragus and the rest of the helix. A postaural fistula into the mastoid is occasionally seen. Inspection of the ear should be carried out with an electric otoscope after selection of a speculum of suitable size. The pinna should be gently but firmly grasped and pulled posteriorly prior to insertion of the speculum. The tympanic membrane should be examined for perforation, thickening or white chalky patches of tympanosclerosis. Wax is a common problem, preventing adequate inspection of the tympanic membrane, and should be removed by syringing with water at 37°C. Before carrying out this procedure it is advisable to investigate the possibility of perforation of the tympanic membrane.

Clinical speech tests

These are useful in order to obtain some information as to how the subject understands the spoken word and is able to discriminate speech. The patient is asked to repeat words spoken to him using a forced whisper and conversational voice at increasing distances from the ear. The ears can be tested separately while a non-tested ear is occluded and masked by pressure on the tragus. In this way an approximation of the degree of hearing loss can be obtained even in the patient's home environment. The examiner will have obtained some insight into the patient's hearing loss in the course of his history taking. Efforts should now be made to test his hearing, using a forced whisper at different distances from each ear after compressing the tragus of the other ear just firmly enough to close the auditory canal. In this way an approximation of the degree of hearing loss and an idea as to which ear is worse affected can be obtained.

Tuning fork methods

A tuning fork at a frequency of 512 Hz is useful in the investigation of patients with hearing disorders. The instrument may be used in the form of two tests:

Weber test

The tuning fork is put into vibration and placed with its base on the midpoint of the vertex of the skull. In a subject with normal hearing the sound of the fork is localized centrally within the head or simultaneously in each ear. In a conductive loss the sound of the tuning fork is heard better in the worse ear, i.e. where there is a conductive hearing defect. In sensorineural hearing loss the sound of the tuning fork is heard better in the good ear.

Rinne test

The tuning fork is placed in front of the ear to assess air conduction and then on the mastoid process to assess bone conduction. If air conduction is better than bone conduction then sensorineural hearing loss is likely.

Conductive hearing loss results in the bone conduction from the mastoid being superior.

Audiogram

The most accurate mode of assessment of the patient's hearing is by means of the audiogram. In this method the minimum loudness in decibels at various frequencies in hertz/Hz is plotted (Fig. 24.1). The hearing levels may be measured by air and bone conduction. In the latter case bone conduction on the contralateral side must be masked to avoid 'crossed' hearing.

In some centres the physician may have access to speech audiometry, in which the degree of hearing loss in regard to the spoken word is measured by adjusting levels of output from a tape recorder.

Tympanometry

In this investigation the acoustical impedance or stiffness of the eardrum is measured. Changes in impedance reflect the condition of the middle ear. The auditory canal is closed with a close-fitting plug in connection with a pump, by which air pressure in the canal can be adjusted. By an acoustical method the degree of stiffness is recorded in the form of a tympanogram.

Acoustic stapedial reflex

This may be used to check for recruitment, which is a feature of sensorineural hearing loss of cochlear origin. When a pure tone signal is applied to the ear, the middle ear muscles of both ears contract. Normally this takes place at a sound level of about 60 dB. The presence of the stapedial reflex is an indicator of a healthy middle ear and undamaged neural structures of the reflex arc, n.VIII and n.VII. When contraction of the ear muscles (stapedius reflex) starts earlier this may point to a process of recruitment.

X-rays

Plain films of the mastoid may show bone erosion, opacity of the middle ear cleft and degree of pneumatization. However, a much more detailed picture of the middle ear, facial nerve and ossicles can be obtained by hypocycloidal polytomography. CT scanning with enhancement is very useful in the diagnosis of small acoustic neuromas.

Electrophysiology

These tests are useful because they are objective, i.e. they do not require the positive cooperation of the patient. This is important in the elderly patient with even minor degrees of dementia which may affect the carrying out of adequate history taking, physical examination and subjective audiometry. Acoustic stimulation may be measured from the brain stem (brain stem evoked responses), and from the cochlea (electrocochleograms).

Calorics and electronystagmography

These are tests of the balancing mechanism and measure responses of the labyrinth to caloric and rotatory stimuli. They record the activity of the integrity of the vestibule and related structures of the inner ear,

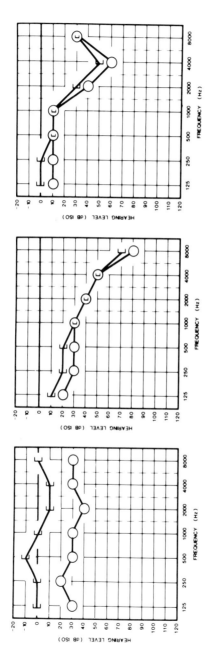

Fig. 24.1 Audiograms from three cases with pathological conditions of the ear. The hearing level in decibels (dB) on the vertical axis is plotted against the frequency of the applied tone on the horizontal axis. In each case bone conduction is shown by a series of square brackets and air conduction by a series of circles. The normal audiogram gives levels of air and bone conduction between zero and 10 dB at all frequencies. The first audiogram on the left shows conductive hearing loss with air conduction alone somewhat reduced. The middle audiogram shows old-age sensorineural hearing loss with both bone and air conduction steadily diminishing towards higher frequencies. The third audiogram is from a case of noise-induced hearing loss. Here, too, there is a deterioration of hearing in both air and bone conduction towards higher frequencies, but there is also a notch at 4000 Hz, which is characteristic for this type of hearing loss

brain stem and higher centres related to the balance mechanism, including eye movements.

DISORDERS OF THE EXTERNAL EAR

Otitis externa

This is very common, and may give rise to conductive hearing loss by constricting the external auditory meatus. On the pinna, frost-bite, chondrodermatitis nodularis helicis — a painful nodule on the helix — and two forms of neoplasm — squamous cell carcinoma and basal cell carcinoma — may be seen. In the external auditory meatus, inflammatory conditions due to viruses (particularly herpes zoster and simplex), bacteria (especially *Staphylococcus aureus* and *Pseudomonas aeruginosa*) and fungi (particularly strains of *Aspergillus*), are also common. Bony osteomata or exostoses may give rise to hearing impairment and are usually associated with cold-water swimming in earlier life.

Attention has been drawn to the existence of minor disturbances of the external auditory meatus in the elderly and which may lead to difficulties in the fitting of hearing aids for the rehabilitation of hearing loss (Maurer & Rupp 1979). Two such conditions are particularly important

1. The most common of these conditions is the presence of a large amount of hardened wax in the external auditory meatus, which may become impacted and lead to conductive hearing loss. It is possible that the reduced tactile sensation that is said to occur in elderly people may result in the subjects not being able to feel the presence of accumulation of wax in the external auditory meatus
2. The other condition is one of prolapsed ear canal caused by loss of elasticity of the cartilage of the external auditory meatus, resulting in a partial, or in rare cases in a complete, dropping of the canal. This may lead to a conduction-type hearing loss and may also cause difficulties in the fitting of moulds for hearing aids

DISORDERS OF THE MIDDLE EAR

Chronic suppurative otitis media

This is a not infrequent finding in the elderly. There may be perforation of the tympanic membrane, polyp formation, tympanosclerosis or cholesteatoma, and operative treatment may be required.

The middle ear is said to manifest a special form of ageing activity with involvement of the joints between the ossicles by arthritic changes and eventual ankylosis. This has been stated to produce in all elderly people a mild degree of hearing loss. However, in an examination of bone and air conduction in approximately 100 elderly subjects in a geriatric hospital I was not able to find any widening of the air–bone gap of any significance. In an additional study of some 20 elderly people for impedance changes I was not able to detect such changes, except in the few cases that showed features of otitis media.

DISORDERS OF THE INNER EAR

Presbyacusis

The commonest cause of deafness in the elderly is presbyacusis, which is a disturbance of cochlear structure and function. There was no understanding of this condition until late in the nineteenth century, when Zwaardemaker in Utrecht (1891) showed that with advancing age hearing of higher frequencies is reduced. By a form of audiometry, using whistles at different pitches, he indicated that the reduction of tone discernment in old age was equivalent to the whole of the uppermost musical octave. He believed it to be a 'labyrinthine' (cochlear) disturbance.

Pathology

Extensive studies of the histological changes found in the temporal bones of the elderly have been made, and various sites in the inner ear may show pathological changes. These include the hair cells (sensory presbyacusis), spiral ganglion cells (neural presbyacusis), stria vascularis (strial or metabolic presbyacusis) and a further type, 'cochlear conductive presbyacusis', which is said to be due to stiffening of the basilar membrane (Schuknecht 1974). Each type of presbyacusis may be associated with its own audiometric feature: sensory presbyacusis with an abrupt high tone loss in the audiogram, neural presbyacusis with a loss of speech discrimination, metabolic presbyacusis with a flat audiometric pattern and cochlear conductive presbyacusis with a straight-line descending audiometric pattern. The concept is an attractive one in allowing the described pathological features of old-age hearing loss to be brought into a single classification, but further carefully documented data would be helpful.

In a pioneering histological study using surface preparations for examining cochlear hair cells, Bredberg (1965) found that outer hair cells were progressively diminished with advancing age. We carried out studies which indicated hair cell damage in all elderly cochleas (Soucek et al 1987). A new technique was devised for sampling, locating and staining the hair cells from the organ of Corti of elderly subjects in

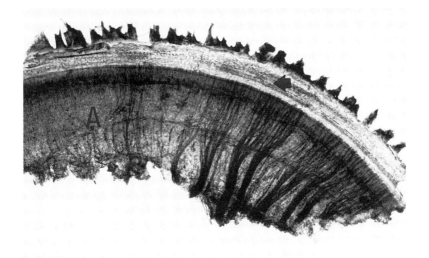

Fig. 24.2 Surface preparation of basal end of cochlea. The surviving organ of Corti and radial nerve fibres are shown to the right of the figure, the organ of Corti region being marked by an arrow. There is almost complete atrophy of the organ of Corti and radial nerve fibres at the extreme basal end at the left (A). Stained by osmic acid and Alcian Blue

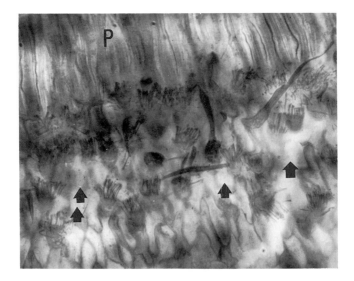

Fig. 24.3 Outer hair cell region of middle coil of cochlea in surface preparation. The stereocilia are seen as clumps of darkly staining thin hairs. Some of them are greatly elongated and thickened to form giant stereocilia, in which the individual component hairs can be seen as dark vertical lines. There are numerous absent hair cells, the position of some of which are marked with arrows. P: pillar cells. Stained with osmic acid and Alcian Blue

whom perilymphatic perfusion with glutaraldehyde or formaldehyde solution had been carried out soon after death. The technique involved microslicing and surface preparations of the undercalcified cochleas. The results of this study allowed us to describe specific pathological changes in the cochlea in presbyacusis.

In 57 cochleas examined by this method the following changes were detected: in all cases, atrophy of the terminal part of the basal coil of the cochlea, including all hair cells and radial nerve fibres; severe loss of outer hair cells and mild loss of inner hair cells throughout the whole cochlea; in all specimens of elderly cochleas severe elongation and fusion of some of the stereocilia of the outer and inner hair cells were present, indicating a specific ageing aberration of the hair cells prior to death (Soucek et al 1987) (Fig. 24.2 and 24.3). The stria vascularis was not affected in these specimens, nor were spiral ganglion cells consistently diminished. These findings explain the general moderate hearing loss and the severe high-frequency hearing loss which are characteristic of presbyacusis.

Clinical and audiological findings

The presenting symptom is usually hearing loss, which may be accompanied by tinnitus. The patient may state that the loss is particularly severe for high tones. Middle ear and central nervous system pathology should be excluded by appropriate clinical examinations. Tuning fork and audiogram investigations confirm the hearing loss particularly at high frequencies.

The patient with presbyacusis may complain of discomfort on hearing a loud noise and this may indicate recruitment. This is a subjective phenomenon in which an ear with sensorineural hearing loss such as in presbyacusis seems to hear tones better than the normal ear. Recruitment may be confirmed by the short increment sensitivity index (SISI) test, in which a short increment of intensity imposed on a carrier tone is used. A carrier tone starting at 20 dB is given 20 increments of 1 dB each, lasting for a fraction of a second. Normal ears will hear only about 20% of the increments. Subjects with presbyacusis usually have almost 100% detection of the increments, indicating a high degree of recruitment and therefore of cochlear damage. Many elderly patients may not be able to concentrate sufficiently for this test and a diagnosis of pure old-age hearing loss may be made on clinical study alone. In doubtful cases brain stem evoked responses may assist in the diagnosis. In presbyacusis the amplitudes of the waves are diminished in this test, but their normal morphology is basically retained. Electrocochleography may also be of value. In this investigation action potentials are of ample proportions, although giving evidence of 'objective recruitment', but cochlear microphonics are markedly reduced owing to reduction of activity of the hair cells (Soucek & Mason 1987) (Fig. 24.4).

Pathogenesis

It has been uncertain whether presbyacusis is of endogenous or exogenous origin, i.e. whether it originates locally in the cochlea as a

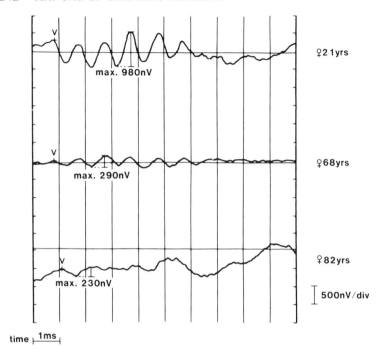

Fig. 24.4 Cochlear microphonic potentials at 80 dB nHL taken from the electrocochleograms of three subjects of 21, 68 and 82 years of age. Note that there is a progressive diminution of the amplitude of the potentials with increasing age

pure ageing phenomenon, or whether it is related to noxious influences from outside the cochlea. Among the latter, excessive noise exposure, hypertension and high blood cholesterol have been suggested as factors in the aetiology of old-age hearing loss in recent years.

In an audiometric investigation of the hearing function of 169 people of average age of about 80 years it was found that all had significant hearing losses, mainly in the higher frequencies, without a history of previous exposure to noise. A further audiometric study of 423 elderly subjects with a variety of medical conditions was undertaken and no specific aetiology could be identified (Souckova 1987). It appears therefore that severe hearing loss in the elderly may occur solely due to age changes in the hair cells of the cochlea.

Noise-induced hearing loss

Awareness of the possibility of noise as the basis of hearing loss in an elderly patient will usually come about in the history taking. The audiogram characteristically shows a notch in the higher tones (Fig. 24.1).

Ototoxicity

Damage to the cochlea from ototoxic drugs is also usually manifested by a sensorineural hearing loss with no other clinical manifestations. Again the history of the patient must be carefully examined to provide evidence for this lesion.

Bone lesions of the otic capsule

Paget's disease of bone frequently affects the bony labyrinth. In some of these cases sensorineural deafness may be the presenting clinical symptom. Examination will reveal the characteristic osseous changes of Paget's, which will be confirmed by radiological investigation and elevation of the serum alkaline phosphatase.

Otosclerosis may present as sensorineural deafness in an elderly subject. This is thought to be the result of involvement of the cochlea by the otosclerotic process. Some evidence of conductive deafness will also be found on audiometry, and radiological features of otosclerosis will be forthcoming.

Acoustic neuroma

A schwannoma of the eighth nerve may be the cause of hearing impairment in a small proportion of elderly patients. There may be concomitant vestibular symptoms such as dizziness. Nystagmus and alteration of the caloric responses will usually support the diagnosis, which will be finalized on the basis of CT scans of the internal auditory meatus.

TINNITUS

About 20% of people over 65 years of age have tinnitus. It is usually intermittent, and only one in 25 is seriously troubled by it.

The cause of tinnitus in the aged is not known, but is thought to be associated with hair cell or neuronal degeneration.

Elderly patients with severe tinnitus find that the noise is worse at night, when surroundings are quiet and less during the day when there is more extraneous sound. This masking effect of external noise may be used by the clinician in treatment and three types of apparatus have been devised and are available for this purpose:

1. Tinnitus maskers, which produce noise at different frequencies and intensities.
2. Hearing aids which by increasing the background noise to ear provide a form of masking.
3. 'Tinnitus instruments': these devices combine the features of a masker with that of a hearing aid.

Such devices alleviate the distress of tinnitus in the long term in about 30% of all tinnitus patients.

Medication is not effective in reducing the loudness or duration of tinnitus. IV lignocaine may relieve the noise for a short period but long-term use is impractical. Psychotherapy, physiotherapy and self-help group therapy offer hope of relief for some subjects. Another approach to the problem is to use electrostimulation to suppress tinnitus and this can be very effective in some subjects. Electrostimulant implants or externally worn units may soon become available. Acupuncture may also give relief in some patients, although this is usually only partial.

HEARING AIDS (Fig. 24.5)

Hearing aids are the mainstay of treatment for the elderly hearing impaired. A hearing aid is a means of applying an increased acoustic pressure on to the tympanic membrane. In the aid an acoustic signal is converted to an electrical signal by a microphone, amplified and filtered and then converted back by the receiver to an acoustic signal. The signal is transmitted through a mould and a tube adapted to the individual external auditory canal. Recent modern improvements in hearing aids allow a range of frequencies from 100 Hz to well over 5000 Hz to be amplified. This includes all of the frequencies that are important for the reception of speech. There are non-directional microphones in use, but

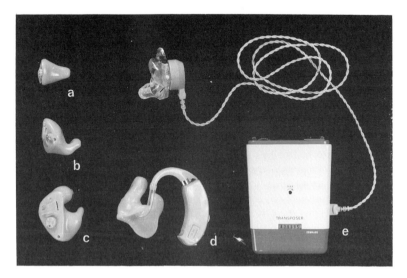

Fig. 24.5 Hearing aids in common use:
(a) canal aid, (b) half concha aid, (c) full concha aid, (d) behind-the-ear aid, and (e) body-worn aid. All photographs at approximately half size (by courtesy of Mr M. Shulberg of Cubex Hearing Centre)

directional microphones are preferable as they allow perception of signal arriving from the front. This provides better speech discrimination. In bone-conduction hearing aids a receiver produces mechanical vibrations. The sound has to be transmitted through the skull and then stimulates the cochlea. This requires much power and output is limited. Bone-conduction hearing aids may be useful where an ear mould cannot be fitted, perhaps due to ear discharge or malformation of the external ear canal.

Hearing aids may be worn in the ear, behind the ear or on the trunk (body-worn). In-the-ear hearing aids are increasingly available. They fit the concha, the external canal, or both. They have the advantages of a microphone within the ear and a good cosmetic effect. The poor handling skills of some elderly people, however, hinders their use. Acoustic feedback can also be a problem if the ear mould does not fit sharply, and is characterized by a high-pitched squeak from the aid.

If the patient requires high amplification a body aid may be required. This aid may also be incorporated into the patient's spectacle frames. Wireless fittings are also possible using FM transmission. Body-worn hearing aids are still used in cases of profound hearing losses. A lead is connected to the box of the hearing aid and the hearing aid receiver. The increased distance between the receiver and microphone minimizes acoustic feedback. This fitting also allows easy handling as the system is robust. The setbacks of body-worn aids are their minimal provision of localizing clues and also the disappearance of higher formants of speech and consonants at certain angles from the speaker which accompanies their use.

Ear moulds

Well-fitting ear moulds are essential if the patient is to derive maximum benefit from the aid. Moulds are made of plastic, and the exact shape is determined by a preliminary impression in silicone of the external ear. In fitting procedures it is vital to obtain a good impression in the first instance. Venting of an ear mould is effective at frequencies below 1 kHz, by allowing these frequencies, which most elderly people hear well, to pass unamplified. In the 1000–3000 Hz region, ear-mould damping is likely to be the primary means of control. Damping appliances using gel-foam are usually inserted in hearing aids to reduce the resonance in the sound transmission channel. Dampers are designed to fit tightly into 2-mm ear-mould tubing; they can be used also at the ear hook or within the hearing aid itself. Horn effects, which control the higher-frequency range above 3000 Hz, can be obtained in hearing aids by adding an attachment such as the 'Libby Horn' to the hearing aid.

Environmental aids to hearing

There are situations where the elderly patient does not benefit from a hearing aid. Here environmental aids to hearing are of value. They include aids designed so that doorbells, alarm clocks, warning devices and telephone amplifiers can be better heard by contact. A hearing aid can also be adapted to an environmental aid such as an external microphone or direct electrical contact with a telephone. A telecommunication device known as a 'deaf communicating terminal' is in use, consisting of a typewriter keyboard and display. Visual or tactile signals converted from audible signals are used in offices, homes or factories. Group conversation is now possible with microphones and amplifiers so that deaf persons can be included. Special doorbells and extensions, alarm clocks and modification of TV amplifying devices are also available.

BIBLIOGRAPHY

Bredberg G (1965) Cellular pattern and nerve supply of the human organ of Corti. Acta Otolaryngologica (suppl) 236: 1–135
Maurer J F, Rupp R R (1979) Hearing and aging. Tactics for intervention. Grace & Stratton, New York
Schuknecht H F (1974) Pathology of the ear. Harvard University Press, Cambridge
Soucek S, Mason S M (1987) A study of hearing in the elderly using non-invasive electrocochleography and auditory brainstem responses. Journal of Otolaryngology 16: 345–353
Soucek S, Michaels L, Frohlich A (1987) Pathological changes in the organ of Corti as revealed by microslicing and staining. Acta Otolaryngologica (suppl)
Souckova S, Soucek S (1987) Investigation of functional and morphological changes in the ear associated with ageing. PhD Thesis, University of London
Zwaardemaker H (1891) Der Verlust an höhen Tonen mit Zunehmendem Alter. Ein neues Gesetz. Archiv für Ohren-Nasen und Hehlkopfheilkunde 32: 53–56

25. BALANCE AND FALLS

CHANGES WITH AGE

Balance

— In normal standing the centre of gravity lies a few centimetres in front of the transverse axis of the ankles. There is a tendency for the body to be pulled forward, which is corrected by contraction of the calf muscles. The continuous movement maintaining the upright posture is called sway

— In addition to the sway response, large forces displacing the centre of gravity are corrected by stepping and tripping reactions or by sweeping movements of the arms

— Postural sway, as measured with an ataxiameter or by other methods, increases with age

— Sway is greater in women than in men at all ages

— Increased sway, greater than that in normal elderly controls, is found in patients who have had non-accidental falls

Gait

Some of the characteristic changes in gait with advancing age are

1. Step length is reduced from 80 cm in young controls to about 65 cm in healthy elderly
2. An increase in the variability of step length
3. The speed of walking is reduced
4. The stride width is increased
5. The period during which the weight of the body is supported on both legs during walking is increased

— The findings are similar to those of normal elderly controls in old people who have fallen due to accidental trips

— Elderly patients admitted to hospital on account of frequent falls show a significant deterioration in all the above gait parameters: step length is increased, walking speed is slower and step length variability is increased. 'Marche à petit pas' is common

FALLS

Epidemiology
— Surveys of a random sample of the elderly population at home indicate that about 20% of men and 40% of women have a history of falls during the previous year (Exton-Smith 1977)
— The proportion who fall increases with age (see Fig. 25.1)
— A decline in the incidence of falls occurs in very old men. This probably represents the survival of an exceptionally fit elite who have characteristics which enable them to outlive their former contemporaries. At one time this phenomenon was thought to be confined to men, but it is now recognized that it also occurs in women 5–10 years later
— The majority of falls at home go unreported. Each year about 3% of old people who fall sustain injuries sufficiently severe to require medical attention
— In residential homes the rate of severe falls is much higher — 11% in one survey (Gryfe et al 1977). This higher rate is in spite of a more protected environment. It presumably reflects the poorer state of health and the frailty of the residents
— In institutions most falls occur within the first week of admission, despite adequate supervision. A low fall rate may indicate low activity and over-protectiveness of the staff

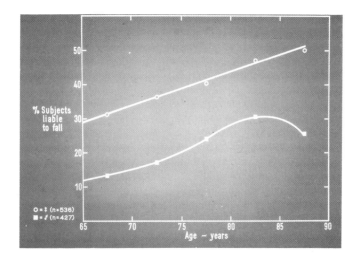

Fig. 25.1 Age incidence of falls

— For old people at home the majority of serious falls occur
during the day in the home or its immediate environs
— Falls on the stairs occur more often when descending

Classification of falls

In the clinical evaluation of falls it is important to obtain an accurate
history of the circumstances of the fall and the events leading up to it.
The history should be augmented by a description from any witness of
the fall.

Trips

— Trips or accidents account for about 45% of all falls.
Typically they occur in people under 75 years who are
active and therefore more likely to sustain accidents
— More old people, in spite of an occasional trip or accident,
tend to maintain their confidence and retain their usual
activities
— Postural sway is not increased and is similar to that in
age-matched controls
— Gait patterns tend to be normal
— After the age of 75 years, although falls due to tripping are
common, the proportion of falls due to this cause declines
and intrinsic factors assume greater importance.

Falls due to intrinsic factors

— These patients are usually unable to explain the
circumstances of their fall. They may say 'I just went
down', 'I lost my balance' or 'I must have had a black-out'
The patient who complains of giddiness rarely has true
vertigo, and in the black-out there is rarely loss of
consciousness to account for the fall
— Multiple aetiological factors are usually responsible for this
type of fall, and there may be defects at several levels in
the systems maintaining balance. Overall there is
considerable reserve and for the patient suffering from
labyrinthine disturbances or cervical spondylosis balance
may still be maintained until he attempts to get out of
bed at night when he is deprived of visual information
— Postural sway is considerably increased in these patients
compared with that in old people who do not fall or in
whom the falls are due to tripping. There is a further
increase in swing when measurements are made with the
eyes closed

Falls following change in position

— Frail elderly people often fall after changes in position, such
as rising from a chair, getting out of bed or moving from a
bed to chair. These activities require the coordinated action

of antigravity muscles if balance is to be maintained
— Postural hypotension can certainly be responsible, but it is rarely found in patients with this type of fall

Spontaneous falls when walking or standing

— The majority of elderly people are able to carry out skilled and well-practised activities without hazard, provided they are not distracted. If, for example, when descending stairs attention is diverted by a telephone or front doorbell ringing, a fall may occur
— If balance is lost there may be great difficulty in recovering due to slowness in reaction, poor coordination of movements, muscle weakness or stiffness of the joints

Drop attacks

— It has been estimated that drop attacks account for 10–25% of falls in the elderly (Overstall et al 1977, Sheldon 1960). They are more common in women than in men but with advancing age the number of men affected increases
— A typical story, for example, is of a woman standing at the kitchen sink peeling potatoes who suddenly finds herself on the floor with the potato in one hand and the knife in the other. There is no loss of consciousness, but the falling to the ground is associated with a complete loss of tone in muscles which maintain the upright posture. Usually the tone returns quickly and the patient is soon able to get up again; there are no neurological sequelae. In other instances the patient remains on the floor. Sometimes recovery in tone is achieved by pressing the soles of the feet against a wall
— The cause of drop attacks is uncertain. Vertebrobasilar insufficiency can probably be responsible: in some patients obstruction to blood flow can be produced in a vertebral artery at the level of the atlanto-occipital membrane by turning the head, or by pressure from osteophytes in cervical spondylosis. But in the majority of patients there is no supporting evidence for brain stem ischaemia
— Several contributing factors are present in most patients and vestibular disorders are invariably found (Hazell 1979). Postural sway is also increased (Overstall et al 1977)

Associated clinical conditions

These may initiate or aggravate falls.

— Acute illness of almost any kind, but especially chest infections, may initiate a fall (premonitory fall)
— Drugs can cause falls in a variety of ways, but most often owing to a slowing of reaction time associated with the use of hypnotics and tranquillizers. Long-acting benzodiazepines lead to hangover effects, confusion or falls; these tend to

become apparent after several weeks administration. Phenothiazines can lead to falls through the production of postural hypotension

— Poor vision has been shown to be an important factor in patients over the age of 75 whose falls lead to fracture of the femoral neck (Brocklehurst et al 1976). Even minor reductions in visual acuity can have a deleterious effect on balance in elderly persons who have deficient afferent information due to defects in other components of the balance system

— Organic brain disease, especially senile dementia of the Alzheimer type, multi-infarct dementia, cerebrovascular disease and parkinsonism, are associated with an increased liability of falls. Elderly patients in psychiatric hospitals have a higher incidence of falls and of fracture of the femoral neck. Elderly fallers have lower mental test scores than age-matched controls

— Vestibular lesions are commoner in those who fall, but are often undetected without special investigation. These patients complain of disequilibrium or unsteadiness, and in some cases true vertigo. Turning the head is blamed by 5% and giddiness by another 9% of old people who fall (Overstall et al 1977). In all these groups postural sway is increased

— Cervical spondylosis is very common in old age and it is likely that it is an important underlying cause of falls. The contribution of the mechanoreceptors in apophyseal joints of the cervical spine is now well recognized. Even in the presence of a normally functioning vestibular system the loss of afferent input from the mechanoreceptors, which occurs in cervical spondylosis, causes vertigo, nystagmus and ataxia. It is more likely that this is the mechanism of falls in cervical spondylosis than vertebrobasilar insufficiency

— Osteoarthritis of the knees, and to a lesser extent of the hips, is an important cause of falls and abnormality of gait. Owing to instability of the knee joints and to loss of muscle tension supporting the joint, falls often occur when descending stairs, and more often than when climbing stairs

— Postural hypotension and syncope are discussed in Chapter 10

Mortality

— Older people who have frequent falls and especially when admission to hospital is required are often in poor health and consequently have a higher mortality than the general elderly population

— One-quarter of old people who have falls due to causes other than tripping die within one year — five times as many as

in a control group without falls. When the fall is due to a
trip the mortality is lower than expected
— Significant factors associated with higher mortality are male
sex, loss of independent mobility due to disorders of gait or
balance, incontinence of urine and mental impairment

Management
— In all old people who fall, attempts should be made to
improve general health and to treat specific clinical
conditions. Harmful drugs must be stopped and particular
attention should be paid to drugs, such as prochlorperazine
which have been prescribed for their 'sedative effect' on the
labyrinth; these agents are more likely to impair balance
than improve it
— Attention should be paid to possible hazards in the
environment, such as loose rugs, trailing flexes, obstacles on
the stairs, defective stair rails, and inadequate lighting of
corridors and stairways
— Apart from attention to safety precautions in the home, fit
old people who trip require no special measures. They
should be urged to resume their usual physical activities
— Patients with poor vision should have their visual acuity
improved if possible by the provision of appropriate
spectacles or by cataract extraction
— Patients whose falls are due to intrinsic factors often lose
confidence, and they may become housebound for fear of
going outside, even though they do not sustain serious
injury in the fall. These patients can often have their
balance improved and confidence restored by appropriate
exercises supervised by the physiotherapist. Exercises which
take about 10 minutes, and should be repeated several times
in the day, have been described by Overstall (1980). The
physiotherapist should also teach the patient how to get up
from the floor should further falls occur

BIBLIOGRAPHY

Brocklehurst J C, Exton-Smith A N, Lempert Barber S M, Hunt L, Palmer M 1976 Fracture
of the femur in old age: A two centre study of associated clinical factors and the cause of
the fall. Age and Ageing 7: 7–15
Exton-Smith A N 1977 Functional consequences of aging: Clinical manifestations, In:
Exton-Smith A N, Evans J G (eds) Care of the elderly: Meeting the challenge of
dependency. Academic Press, London. pp 41–57
Gryfe C I, Amies A, Ashley M J 1977 A longitudinal study of falls in an elderly population.
Age and Ageing 6: 201–211
Hazell J W P 1979 Vestibular problems of balance. Age and Ageing 8: 258–260
Overstall P W 1980 Prevention of falls in the elderly. Journal of the American Geriatrics
Society 28: 481–484

Overstall P W, Imms F, Exton-Smith A N, Johnson A L 1977 Falls in the elderly related to
     postural imbalance. British Medical Journal 1: 261–264
Sheldon J H 1960 On the natural history of falls in old age. British Medical Journal
     2: 1685–1690

26. URINARY INCONTINENCE

NORMAL BLADDER FUNCTION

Anatomy, physiology and pharmacology

— A diagrammatic representation of the male and female lower urinary tract is shown in Figures 26.1 and 26.2
— The bladder should normally store a urine volume of about 500 ml without leaking. When micturition becomes appropriate the detrusor muscle should develop a sustained coordinated contraction associated with a sustained relaxation of the sphincter and urethra
— The pharmacology of the receptors in the lower urinary tract is shown in Table 26.1

Table 26.1 Receptor pharmacology

Site	Type	Function
Detrusor muscle	Parasympathetic efferents S2, 3, 4 Mainly cholinergic. A few $\beta2$ and $\alpha1$ receptors from hypogastric nerves	Voiding
Internal sphincter	Mainly $\alpha1$ receptors	Excitatory
	Some cholinergic receptors	Excitatory
Smooth muscle of urethra	$\beta2$ receptors	Inhibitory
Prostatic capsule	Mainly $\alpha1$, few cholinergic	Excitatory
	Few $\beta2$	Inhibitory
External sphincter	Cholinergic, ?α adrenergic	Excitatory
Urethra (female)	Oestrogen (especially distal two-thirds)	Maintains urethral function

MALE

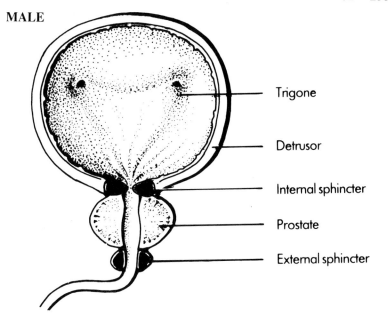

Trigone

Detrusor

Internal sphincter

Prostate

External sphincter

Fig. 26.1

FEMALE

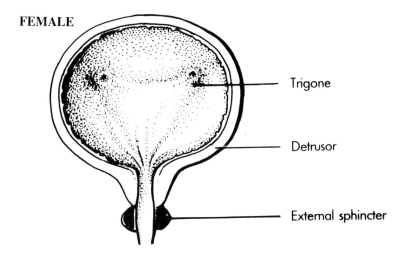

Trigone

Detrusor

External sphincter

Fig. 26.2

Central nervous system control

— The cerebral cortical micturition centre is located in the
superomedial aspects of the frontal lobes adjacent to the
corpus callosum. It receives information from the ascending
sensory pathways and from the brain-stem nuclei. Efferents
leave on association fibres, commisural fibres or descend to
the brain-stem nuclei or the spinal tracts. Electrical
stimulation of the cortical micturition centre produces
detrusor activity

— In the pons and medulla there are motor nuclei concerned
with detrusor activity. Stimulation of these nuclei causes
precipitant detrusor activity and ablation causes inactivity

— From the brain-stem motor nuclei the descending fibres are
organized in three main tracts

  • Nerves originating in the pons, medulla and mid-brain
    pass into the lateral spinoreticular tract to the motor
    nuclei of the sacral cord. Stimulation causes a sustained
    contraction of the detrusor with inhibition of the smooth
    and striated muscle sphincters

  • A second group of fibres descends from the pons in the
    medial reticulospinal tract and function to inhibit the
    striated sphincter

  • Nerves in the third group arise in the medulla and
    descend in the anterior reticulospinal tract and function
    to inhibit the detrusor and to stimulate the sphincters

— Fibres in the medial reticulospinal tract probably synapse
with a unique group of cells (Onuff cells) in the medial
portion of the venterolateral aspect of the anterior horn of
segments S2 and S3. They consist of a mixture of motor
neuron and autonomic cells and probably innervate the
external sphincter of the urethra and the anal sphincter

— Afferent inputs to the central nervous system from the
bladder and urethra originate mainly from the tension
receptors. The receptors respond to distension or
contraction of the bladder but thresholds vary. The afferents
which pass to the sacral region of the cord respond to low
bladder volumes. From about two-thirds bladder capacity
they form a short local reflex arc which inhibits the detrusor
muscle, thereby allowing filling of the bladder without rise
in pressure

— Sacral afferents also form another reflex arc which is
essential for voiding; they synapse with motor nerves either
at the sacral level or, more importantly, after ascending in
the lateral dorsal columns to the brain stem. These reflex
arcs are modified by the influence of neurons from the
higher centres and when uninhibited voiding is initiated

— Afferents from tension receptors located mainly in the muscle coats and the submucosa of the bladder neck and the urethra reach the central nervous system by the lumbar segments of the cord. They respond to extreme pressure and start functioning at larger bladder volumes

MECHANISMS OF INCONTINENCE

Detrusor instability

This condition is due to damage to the descending fibres carrying inhibitory impulses. The symptoms are frequency, nocturia, urgency and urge incontinence.

Unsustained detrusor activity

Damage to pathways responsible for voiding leads to the development of a chronic residual urine which, when it becomes infected, aggravates any existing instability.

Detrusor sphincter dyssynergia

Damage to the descending pathways can also affect coordination between sphincter relaxation and detrusor contraction. The symptoms are hesitancy and a reduction in urine stream, together with problems due to a chronic residual volume.

Hypotonic bladder

This condition results from damage to the sacral cord or the peripheral nerves supplying the bladder and urethra. The typical symptoms are a recurrent urinary tract infection associated with the high residual volume, persistent dribbling incontinence and precipitant incontinence. A strong indication of hypotonia is incontinence precipitated by standing. Acute retention is a late sequel. Apart from sacral cord lesions the commonest cause is diabetes mellitus; other evidence of autonomic neuropathy may be found in diabetic patients with hypotonic bladder.

Stress incontinence

Damage resulting from childbirth or urethral instrumentation can lead to impairment of the functional efficiency of the urethra which may be further impaired by oestrogen lack in later life. The diagnosis can be made by examining the patient while standing, the bladder full and asking her to cough. It must be borne in mind that coughing, laughing and other stresses can induce unstable contractions in patients with detrusor instability, which may therefore masquerade as stress incontinence. Indeed, the two conditions may coexist.

Overflow incontinence

Obstructive lesions of the outflow tract, such as prostatism and strictures, may lead to incontinence. But most patients with prostatic enlargement have voiding difficulties or complete retention without developing incontinence. Patients with outflow obstruction, however, do complain of frequency and urgency. This is probably due to the detrusor muscle becoming hyperactive in response to the obstruction. Surgical correction of the obstruction will lead to return of normal function of the detrusor. Surgical intervention will not influence the unstable contractions when detrusor instability existed before the development of obstruction.

> — A very high proportion of incontinent patients have several functional disturbances; the presence of multiple aetiological factors is the rule rather than the exception. Detrusor instability and hypotonia are not mutually exclusive since the two often coexist. When a voiding problem leads to a rising residual volume the excessive stretching of the detrusor muscle produces a hypotonic bladder

INCONTINENCE IN NEUROLOGICAL DISEASES

Incontinence is an important feature of many neurological diseases.

Dementia of the Alzheimer type

Detrusor instability and unsustained detrusor contractions are often the result of dementia. The characteristic pattern in these patients is repetitive micturition behaviour. Owing to their mental impairment the patients have a lack of insight into their condition.

Cerebrovascular disease

This condition commonly produces detrusor instability. Many of the patients have a voiding problem either because detrusor contraction is unsustained or because of sphincter dyssynergia. In the incontinence which follows a stroke the main contributing factors are mental impairment, previous moderate or severe motor deficit and current reduction in mobility. Dysphasia in patients with right hemiplegia is associated with incontinence; the patient is unable to summon help and make his needs known. Parietal lobe involvement in those with left hemiplegia is not associated with incontinence. The prognosis is good in patients whose orientation, mobility and ability for self-care improve.

Parkinsonism

Detrusor instability is found in the early stages. Later, further functional disturbances develop; a voiding problem occurs when detrusor contractions become less sustained and this eventually evolves into frank hypotonia. Shy–Drager syndrome, with or without parkinsonian features, almost invariably produces incontinence.

Multiple sclerosis

Because of its progressive nature several disturbances occur. Detrusor instability is usually an early feature, to be followed by a voiding problem due to unsustained detrusor activity or to dyssynergia. In multiple sclerosis and in the above-mentioned neurological diseases the bladder disturbances tend to evolve.

PREVALENCE OF INCONTINENCE

— Surveys of the elderly population show that approximately 7% of men and 12% of women over the age of 70 are incontinent. In the age group 15–64 years the prevalence is 1.6% of men and 7% of men and 12% of women over the age of 60 years
— An even greater prevalence of incontinence is found in old people in residential homes and elderly patients in hospital, where surveys show that 15–50% are incontinent. The highest prevalence is found in psychogeriatric units

INVESTIGATION OF THE INCONTINENT PATIENT

— The majority of patients can be assessed by an algorithmic approach which does not require complex investigation. This method, which has been described by Hilton & Stanton (1981), has proved to be effective
— In order to assess voiding efficiency in patients with suspected hypotonic bladder it is necessary to measure the residual urine volume after micturition by passing a Jacques catheter
— The most thorough investigation of incontinence which is needed in some patients is best achieved by pressure/flow

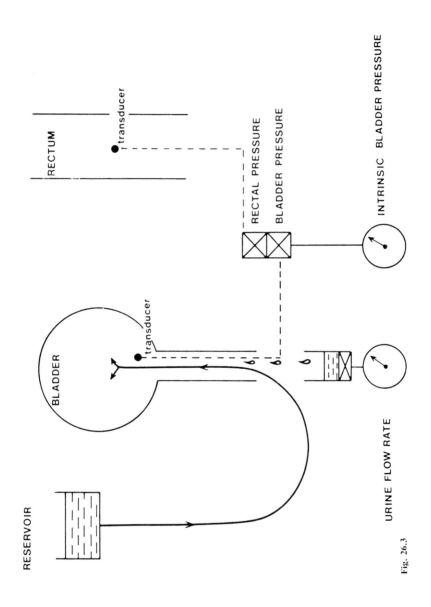

Fig. 26.3

cystometry or by videocystometry (Turner-Warwick & Whiteside 1979). Dynamic investigations are essential to elucidate the relative importance of the different functional disturbances which often coexist. Rational treatment can only be practised on the basis of accurate assessment
— A diagrammatic representation of a urodynamic study is shown in Figure 26.3
— Urodynamic investigations are not difficult to carry out and the technique is available in most incontinence clinics. The interpretation of the findings, however, requires considerable experience. For a further description of voiding studies, see Malone-Lee (1985)

Management

Although in this section the management of each type of disturbance of function will be described, it is important to view the situation as a whole owing to the coexistence of several aetiological factors. The management of detrusor instability and hypotonia, for example, requires a balance of opposing therapies.

Detrusor instability
— The treatment of this condition is most satisfactorily achieved by a bladder-retraining regimen, the aim of which is to stretch the detrusor and so reduce its activity. The patient keeps a simple bladder record chart and is encouraged to increase the interval between each micturition. It is usually found that once a minimum interval of 4 hours is attained the symptoms due to instability lessen. During the retraining programme the patient should be followed up regularly at 2-weekly intervals
— Drug therapy should be considered at the start of the retraining programme
  • Imipramine, a tricyclic antidepressant, has anticholinergic agonist and anti-5-HT actions. The response to treatment is often good using a dose of 10–25 mg nocte
  • Propantheline is a quaternary ammonium compound with muscarinic blocking actions. Its action on detrusor instability is unpredictable, probably due to its irregular absorption from the gastrointestinal tract
  • Oxybutynin is an antispasmodic with a papaverine action. Although this drug is often effective it has limited use because of side effects, in particular an extremely dry mouth
  • Emepronium bromide (Cetiprin) is now out of licence. It should not be used because of its variable efficiency due to irregular absorption. Oesophageal ulceration is a troublesome side effect
  • Terodoline is a secondary amine with anticholinergic effects together with a calcium antagonistic effect. It is

well absorbed from the gut and well tolerated, apart from the production of dry mouth. Several placebo-controlled studies have shown its effectiveness in a dose of 37.5–50 mg daily. Improvement occurs in both symptoms and cystometric measurements (Drugs and Therapeutics Bulletin, 1988)

Voiding problems

— Patients with functional voiding problems can usually be greatly helped by intermittent catheterization. The residual urine should be removed with a Jacques catheter at a frequency of two to three times a day. It is even possible for the patient to carry out the procedure at home using a clean non-sterile technique. It is often successful in re-establishing normal voiding. Cholinergic drugs for the long-term treatment of voiding problems have proved of little value

— When the voiding problem is due to organic obstruction this must be dealt with surgically

Sphincter incompetence

— This, too, may require surgical correction. Minor urethral lesions may respond to pelvic exercises, which can be supplemented with low-dose oestrogen therapy applied locally

Irreversible incontinence

— There are some patients whose incontinence is unresponsive to treatment and their management must depend on incontinence aids. For comprehensive descriptions of such appliances, suitable clothing and their sources of supply the reader is referred to the publication of the Disabled Living Foundation (Elphick 1970) and the booklet by Dorothy Mandelstam (1977)

— During the past decade advances have been made in the development of absorbents. The newer body-worn disposable pads are now proving much more effective. Patients have very different requirements and the garment system must be chosen to suit the individual (Malone-Lee et al 1983)

— A permanent indwelling catheter may produce more problems than it solves. When catheterization is used as a last resort the catheter should be of small-gauge silicone with a small balloon. Urinary tract infection should be treated only when there are symptoms. Bladder washouts should be reserved for those whose catheter becomes blocked repeatedly

BIBLIOGRAPHY

Drugs and Therapeutics Bullentin 1988 Terodoline and oxybutyrin in detrusor instability.
26: 37–38

Elphick L 1970 Incontinence. Disabled Living Foundation, London

Exton-Smith A N, Weksler M E (eds) 1985 Practical geriatric medicine. Churchill Livingstone,
Edinburgh

Hilton P, Stanton S L 1981 Algorithmic method of assessing urinary incontinence in elderly
women. British Medical Journal 282: 940–942

Malone-Lee J G 1985 Urinary incontinence. In: Exton-Smith A N, Weksler M Practical
geriatric medicine. Churchill Livingstone, Edinburgh

Malone-Lee J G, McCreery M, Exton-Smith A N 1983 A community study of incontinence
garments. Report of the Department of Health and Social Security, HMSO, London

Mandelstam D 1977 Incontinence. Heinemann, London

Sheldon J H 1948 The social medicine of old age. Nuffield Foundation, Oxford University
Press, Oxford

Thomas T M, Flymat K R, Blannin J, Meade T W 1980 Prevalence of urinary incontinence.
British Medical Journal 281: 1243–1245

Turner-Warwick R, Whiteside C G (eds) 1979 Clinical urodynamics. Urologic Clinics of North
America 6: 1

27. ACCIDENTAL HYPOTHERMIA

Definition

A hypothermic state exists when the deep body temperature falls below an arbitrarily defined limit of 35.0°C. The term accidental is used to imply that the hypothermia occurs unintentionally, i.e. not necessarily associated with a fall or other accident.

— Primary hypothermia occurs when exposure to cold is solely or chiefly responsible. In the elderly there is often 'physiological' impairment of temperature regulation, not associated with obvious disease

— Secondary hypothermia is present when the hypothermia is a manifestation of underlying disease, although the low body temperature is often precipitated by cold exposure

Diagnosis

The diagnosis can only be made by the use of a low-reading clinical or electronic thermometer (25–40°C). Rectal temperature measurement is the method of choice; oral temperature recordings are misleading, especially in low environmental temperatures.

Aetiology

— Multiple aetiological factors are often responsible
  - Exposure to cold
  - Low metabolic heat production
  - Impaired thermoregulation
  - Impaired shivering thermogenesis
  - Impaired temperature perception
  - Disease
  - Drugs

— Cold exposure is an overriding factor in primary hypothermia and is often present in secondary hypothermia. A common story is of an old person who falls after getting out of bed at night; he remains on the floor for several hours, often partly clad, and is discovered only the next day by a neighbour or home help. Thus exposure is usually longer when the patient lives alone or is socially isolated

— Low metabolic heat production is particularly important in the elderly. Hypothermia can occur with comparatively mild degrees of cold exposure, e.g. when the old person is in bed at night, apparently well covered. Insufficient body heat is being generated, so that even good external insulation is ineffective

— Impaired temperature regulation is an important factor responsible for the high incidence of accidental hypothermia in the old. Owing to physiological decline in thermoregulatory capacity the normal difference (4.5–5.0°C) between the deep (core) and the superficial (shell) temperatures cannot be maintained owing to reduced vasoconstriction in response to cold

— Impaired shivering thermogenesis is a notable factor affecting temperature in many old people. It has been demonstrated in apparently normal 80-year-olds and in those who have recovered from an episode of hypothermia. Using a body cooling unit Collins et al (1981) have compared the metabolic response to cooling in the healthy elderly and in young control subjects. Shivering was absent or less intense in the older group and the increase in metabolic heat production was significantly less than in young controls

— Impaired thermal perception is responsible for diminished sensitivity to cold shown by many old people. Whereas younger people can detect temperature differences as small as 0.5°C using tests or digital thermosensation, older people may not be able to detect differences as large as 5.0°C or

Table 27.1 Common clinical conditions associated with hypothermia

Endogenous disorders
Myxoedema and hypopituitarism
Diabetes mellitus (numerically more important, especially in those with autonomic neuropathy)

Neurological disorders
Cerebrovascular accident causing a fall, leading to cold exposure
Paralysis with limitation of heat production
Parkinsonism, in which autonomic impairment may be present
Autonomic neuropathy (see Ch. 19)

Conditions causing immobility
Stupor or coma due to various causes
Paraplegia
Parkinsonism
Severe arthritis

Mental impairment
Dementia: if the patients are receiving insufficient care and supervision they are at special risk of cold exposure

Severe infections and circulatory disturbances
Bronchopneumonia
Septicaemia
Cardiac infarction

more. In consequence many old people appear to be able to tolerate cold conditions without discomfort; but because they are unaware of the cold they fail to take the necessary protective action to shield them against it, and they may be at risk of over-taxing a failing thermoregulatory system

— Diseases become of greater importance with increasing age. Most cases of hypothermia admitted to hospital have one or more clinical conditions. The more common of these are shown in Table 27.1, but almost any serious disorder can lead to hypothermia

— The main drugs affecting temperature regulation and likely to lead to hypothermia under cold conditions are
  • Phenothiazines
  • Antidepressants
  • Hypnotics
  • Alcohol

Clinical features

— The patient usually has a grey colour due to a mixture of pallor and cyanosis. The skin is cold to the touch, not only in exposed parts of the body but also in those parts normally covered, such as the axillae and abdominal wall. The puffy facial appearance, the slow cerebration and a husky voice may be mistaken for myxoedema

— An acute confusional state is often a salient feature. Drowsiness increases as the temperature falls. In the series reported by Rosin & Exton-Smith (1964) three-quarters of the patients with rectal temperatures below 27°C were unconscious

— Shivering is usually absent and is replaced by muscular hypertonus which gives rise to neck stiffness simulating meningism and to rigidity of the abdominal wall. In some patients an involuntary flapping tremor occurs (Rosin and Exton-Smith, 1964)

— The heart rate slows due to sinus bradycardia or slow atrial fibrillation. The ECG usually shows some degree of heart block with lengthening of the PR interval in patients with sinus rhythm. A pathognomonic sign is a J-wave shown by a characteristic deflection at the junction of the QRS and ST segments. The size of the wave is not related to the severity of the hypothermia; indeed, in some cases the J-wave is absent altogether, even in severe hypothermia

— In severe hypothermia the respirations are slow and shallow which can progress to apnoea. The pO_2 in the arterial blood is low, and the oxygen dissociation curve is shifted so that less oxygen is given up to the tissues. The consequent tissue anoxia may be an important factor influencing prognosis. Bronchopneumonia may be present

without the usual clinical signs, and the basal crepitations may be due to cold injury to the alveoli
— Acute pancreatitis is often found at post-mortem examination but during life it is often overlooked since few of the typical signs are present in the hypothermic patient. It should be suspected if the patient winces when pressure is applied to the epigastrium. A rise in the serum amylase is found in the majority of cases of severe hypothermia
— Renal blood flow and glomerular filtration rate are decreased and tubular function is impaired. Oliguria is common and acute tubular necrosis can occur. This may be due to a combination of ischaemia and the direct effect of cold on the kidneys

The temperatures at which clinical manifestations generally appear are shown in Table 27.2, but there is great variability.

Table 27.2   Accidental hypothermia; clinical manifestations

Core temperature (°C)	Signs
37	Normal temperature responses
36	Peripheral vasoconstriction Shivering
35	Clinical hypothermia
34–33	Impaired coordination Slow cerebration Confusion
32–31	Drowsiness Slow heart rate Slow respiration
30–29	Muscular hypertonus (neck stiffness and rigidity of limbs) Flapping tremor ± ECG: Sinus bradycardia Slow atrial fibrillation Prolonged PR interval J waves ±
28–27	Increased myocardial irritability Risk of ventricular fibrillation Absent tendon reflexes Fall in blood pressure Vascular thromboses Pancreatitis
26–24	Ventricular fibrillation Pulmonary oedema
20–17	Cardiac standstill ECG — isoelectric

Management

In many cases of mild hypothermia (34–35°C) not associated with serious illness the temperature will rise spontaneously when the patient is moved to warmer conditions. Careful monitoring of the rectal temperature every half to one hour is necessary. In moderate and severe cases the therapeutic regimens outlined in Table 27.3 should be adopted.

Table 27.3 Management of accidental hypothermia

Mild to moderate hypothermia (32–34°C)
  Nurse in cubicle maintained at 25–30°C
  Allow core temperature to rise at 0.5°C per hour
  Barrier nursing; administer broad-spectrum antibiotic
  Oxygen administration through Venturi mask
  Pulse and blood pressure monitoring continuously or half-hourly
  If possible treat associated clinical conditions
  Active measures for the prevention of pressure sores

Severe hypothermia (below 32°C)
Additional measures to the above:
  Treatment in intensive care unit
  Institute positive pressure ventilation
  Insert central venous catheter to monitor pressure and to administer warm fluids
  Correct dehydration and electrolyte disturbances
  IV prophylactic antibiotic, e.g. cloxacillin
  Monitor core temperature continuously, e.g. by thermistor in external auditory meatus or by rectal thermometer
  Continous blood pressure monitoring; if blood pressure falls recool patient
  ECG monitoring for arrythmias

Prognosis

The prognosis is good if the general condition of the patient is satisfactory and if the underlying cause (e.g. drugs) can be removed. It is poor if

— Hypothermia is severe
— Duration of hypothermia is prolonged
— Complications develop (e.g. circulatory collapse with fall in blood pressure)
— Underlying disease cannot be corrected

Preventive measure

— Recognizing those at risk
  • Doctors and community nurses should pay particular attention to old people living in cold conditions, even though they do not complain of the cold
  • Deep body temperatures should be regularly recorded of old people whose activities are restricted by chronic illness or disability
  • Social workers should look for unmet needs in isolated old people
— Heating
  • So far as it is possible install safe and convenient

methods of heating (e.g. central heating or night storage heating)

- Improve the thermal insulation of the dwelling by loft insulation and eliminating draughts
- In severe conditions keep the living room warm and move the bed into it
- Wider publicity is needed to make known to old people the availability of an extra heating allowance for those in receipt of income support

— Clothing and blankets

- For maximum comfort and warmth clothing should be light, closely woven and not restricting
- The same considerations apply to bed clothes. A woollen cap worn at night minimizes heat loss through the head, which can be considerable
- Since many cases of hypothermia occur at night the risks can be reduced but not eliminated by the use of an electric blanket. This should be either an over-blanket or a low-voltage, low-wattage under-blanket (especially important in incontinent patients)

— Nutrition

- Many of the factors which lead to hypothermia also lead to malnutrition, so the two conditions often occur together
- The cost of keeping warm in winter may leave insufficient money for food. Many pensioners are on the borderline of malnutrition, which may become overt when the energy needs of the body are highest
- The provision of meals on wheels for those at risk and especially the housebound is a valuable preventive measure and helps to keep otherwise healthy old people under the supervision of the social services
- Lean old people are at greater risk because they lack adequate subcutaneous tissue which prevents heat loss, but they are usually more active. The obese elderly, although better protected, are also at risk because they tend to be less active
- Alcohol consumption should be restricted since, although inducing an internal sensation of warmth, it produces vasodilatation and promotes heat loss

BIBLIOGRAPHY

Fox R H, Woodward P M, Exton-Smith A N, Green M F, Donnison D V, Wicks M H 1973 Body temperatures in the elderly: A national study of physiological, social and environmental conditions. British Medical Journal 1: 200

Collins K J 1983 Hypothermia: The facts. Oxford University Press, Oxford

Collins K J, Easton, J, Exton-Smith A N 1981 Shivering thermogenesis and vasomotor responses with convective cooling in the elderly. Proceedings of the Physiological Society 320: 76

Collins K J, Exton-Smith A N 1983 Thermal homeostasis in old age. Journal of the American Geriatrics Society 31: 519–524

Maclean D, Emslie-Smith D 1977 Accidental hypothermia. Blackwell Scientific Publications, Oxford

Rosin A, Exton-Smith A N 1964 Clinical features of accidental hypothermia with observations on thyroid function. British Medical Journal 1: 16–19

28. PAIN

- Pain has been defined by the International Association for the Study of Pain (IASP) as an unpleasant sensory and emotional experience associated with actual or potential tissue damage or described in terms of such damage
- Like all sensations it has a threshold which varies not only from person to person but also with time in the same individual. The factors which can affect the threshold include intrinsic personality and cultural background, as well as anxiety, fear, depression, sleep deprivation and isolation. Therefore treatment of pain needs to take into consideration the presence or absence of these factors as well as the severity and the type of pain

Anatomy and physiology
- Pain as a sensation is appreciated by three types of pain receptors (nociceptors), which are small myelinated and unmyelinated nerve fibres
  1. A delta nociceptor, which is distributed fairly superficially on the body surface and is sensitive to high-intensity mechanical stimuli
  2. Nociceptors with myelinated fibres which are present in the deeper part of the skin and are said to be sensitive to mechanical, thermal and chemical stimuli
  3. c-Polymodal nociceptors are 'free nerve endings' which themselves act as receptors
- The nerve fibres from the receptors enter the spinal cord and make connection in the grey matter. The nerve fibres from the delta nociceptors end in lamina I; the nerve fibres from the deeper part of the skin end in lamina V as well as in the dorsal horn lamina, and fibres from c-polymodal nociceptors end in lamina II.
- The fibres travel via the spinothalamic tract, through the reticular formation and intralaminar thalamus to the cortex, predominantly to the prefrontal region.
- At the spinal cord level it is postulated that there is a 'gate' which allows the pain stimuli to pass through to a higher level. It is influenced not only by higher centres but by the

type of fibres stimulated. The stimulation of small fibres tends to open the 'gate', while the stimulation of large-diameter 'A' fibres tends to close the 'gate'

Treatment

Analgesics

— Treatment of pain requires accurate and full assessment of the patient, including his mental and psychological state
— Therapy (Table 28.1) should start with mild analgesics such as aspirin or paracetamol. If, however, these fail to control pain or if the patient develops side effects, he or she should be given dihydrocodeine or dextropropoxyphene. Non-steroidal anti-inflammatory agents may also be tried for mild to moderate degrees of pain, particularly if the pain is due to inflammatory arthritis or to bone disease

Table 28.1 Therapeutic agents used to control pain

For mild pain	Aspirin 300–900 mg tds Paracetamol 1 g 4–6-hourly
For mild to moderate pain	Dextropropoxyphene 65 mg 6–8-hourly (usually given in a compound preparation) Dihydrocodeine 30–60 mg, 6-hourly
For pain due to arthritis or bone disease	Naprosyn 250–500 mg bd Flurbiprofen 100 mg bd Indomethacin 25–50 mg tds
For moderate to severe pain	Buprenorphine 0.4 mg 6–8-hourly sublingually Morphine or diamorphine given orally, by IM injection or by SC infusion pump MST continuous (slow-release preparation), starting dose 10–30 mg bd. The dose is increased until satisfactory response is achieved

— For moderate to severe degree of pain, particularly due to malignant disease process, opiates should be considered. These can be given orally, sublingually, subcutaneously by slow infusion or in a slow-release preparation. Adequate dosage should be given at regular intervals to secure pain control without producing drowsiness or other side effects
— In some patients with moderate to severe degree of pain, analgesics may have to be given with an antidepressant or phenothiazine to potentiate the analgesic effect as well as to control the anxiety related to pain
— In patients with cancer pain one should not worry about psychological dependence or tolerance. The latter in fact develops very slowly and can be matched by small dose increases
— For the side effects of treatment, such as nausea and vomiting, the patient may have to be given prochloperazine

5 mg 4–8-hourly or metoclopamide 10 mg tds. To treat constipation due to dihydrocodeine or other opiates, the patient should be given lactulose
— Sedation with strong opiates is usually mild and self-limiting. The nightmares or hallucinations due to morphine may require haloperidol

Other methods of treatment
In addition to pharmacotherapy for pain, there are many physical and other means of treating pain, and these include those listed in Table 28.2 (some with the contraindications):

Table 28.2

Treatment	Contraindications
Heat-direct or by indirect method such as microwaves, short waves, etc.	Impaired sensation Haemorrhage Acute inflammation/sepsis Trauma
Cryotherapy	Ischaemia Healing wound History of Raynaud's disease
Hydrotherapy	
Ultrasound — may also produce heat by oscillation of particles	Malignancy Acute infection Thrombophlebitis
Transcutaneous electrical nerve stimulation	Cardiac pacemaker
Irradiation — particularly useful for localized malignant deposit	
Nerve block Lumbar sympathectomy Plexus block Continuous epidural infusion Acupuncture	

Treatment of special types of pain
— Pain due to polymyalgia rheumatica/giant cell arteritis responds well to prednisolone
— Pain due to trigeminal neuralgia may respond to chlorpromazine, carbamazepine or phenytoin
— Post-hemiplegic thalamic pain is usually very difficult to control but in some patients it may respond to carbamazepine or phenothiazine
— Pain due to raised intracranial pressure responds to dexamethasone

BIBLIOGRAPHY

Nuki G 1983 Non-steroidal analgesic and anti-inflammatory agents. British Medical Journal 287: 39–43

Wall D, Metzack R (eds) 1984 Textbook of pain. Churchill Livingstone Edinburgh

Page C M 1988 Terminal care at home. Prescribers Journal 28: 8–13

Wells P E, Frampton V, Bowser D (eds) 1988 Pain—management and control in physiotherapy. Heinemann, London

29. PRESSURE SORES

Pressure sores (decubitus ulcers) become increasingly common with advancing age. Elderly patients are so prone to develop sores that the problems of their prevention have a most pertinent connection with the practice of geriatric medicine. If we are to treat diseases in old age we must prevent the damaging effect on the tissues of sustained pressure over localized areas of the body.

Incidence and sites

— Several studies have shown (Norton et al 1962, Barbenel et al 1977, Hibbs 1982) the progressive rise in incidence with age. In a one-day census of a district general hospital in inner London (Hibbs 1982), including medical, surgical, orthopaedic, geriatric and psychiatric beds, 25% required special care for the prevention and management of pressure sores (10% of those under 70 years and 40% over this age)
— Common sites are
  • The sacrum (40%)
  • The heels (20%)
  • The ischial tuberosities (15%)
  • Hips (10%)

Types of sore

— Superficial sore (80%); necrosis is confined to the skin. It often starts as a blister, which breaks down to expose a flat, painful, raw area
— Deep or gangrenous sore (20%); necrosis involves subcutaneous tissue. Damage in the deep tissues is greater than in the skin, so that the sores have overhanging edges

Pathogenesis

Intrinsic and extrinsic factors
The most important factors are
  — The condition of the patient
    • Physical and mental state

- Particular aspects of the condition
— Nursing care
  - Measures used for the relief of pressure
  - Frequency and standard of care
  - Local applications
— Factors surrounding the patient
  - Manner of nursing the patient
  - Material of the mattress, drawsheet, etc.
  - Contact of urine and faeces
  - Infection

Whatever the relative contribution of these components the most important factor is pressure transmitted through the skin and subcutaneous tissue in those regions overlying bony prominences. Pressure when sustained long enough leads to obliteration of blood vessels, ischaemia and necrosis of tissue.

Pressure effects on the tissues

— In experimental animals it has been shown that the skin is more resistant to pressure than subcutaneous tissue or muscle
— Force is distributed over a wide area of skin but tends to be concentrated within a small area where subcutaneous tissue or muscle overlies bony prominences (see Fig. 29.1). Since it is here that the pressure is greatest, and possibly as much as seven times higher than the interface pressure at the skin surface, pressure sores start in the deep tissues. Irreparable and extensive damage may have occurred at a time when the skin only shows erythema

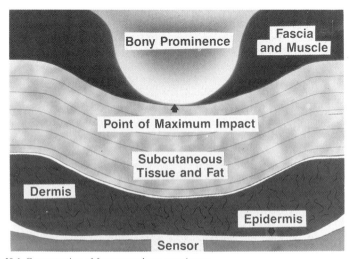

Fig. 29.1 Concentration of forces over bony prominence.

— Low pressure maintained for long periods is often more damaging than high pressure for short periods, i.e. the duration of pressure is just as important as its intensity. In animal experiments, using both normal and denervated muscle, it has been shown that there is an inverse relationship between the intensity and duration of pressure which can be tolerated before pathological changes are noted
— Microscopic changes in muscle occur after a critical time interval of between 1 or 2 hours. It has also been shown that there is a greater resistance to change following the application of equal amounts of alternating pressure (Kosiak 1961)

Compression and shearing forces

There are two main ways in which tissue damage can be produced
— Compression (direct pressure) of tissues which lie between supporting surface and the nearest bony prominence (see Fig. 29.1)
— Shearing forces are responsible for damage particularly over the sacrum and the heels. When the head of the bed is raised by a few inches or when the patient is nursed in a semi-recumbent position, a shearing force is exerted at these sites. If the friction between the skin and the underlying surface is the only force opposing the body slipping down in bed, the loosely attached superficial tissues slide over the

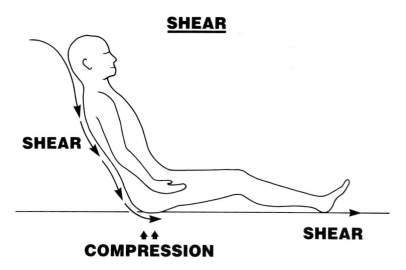

Fig. 29.2 Shearing forces over sacral area.

well-anchored deep fascia through which the blood vessels
pass to the skin.

Vessels may be kinked, obliterated or ruptured. The consequent tissue
necrosis leads to an appearance which differs from that due to direct
compression and a large amount of undermining extends circumferentially
around the base of the ulcer.

Evaluation of clinical factors

Clinical condition of the patients

- Pressure of sufficiently long duration to cause tissue damage
  rarely occurs in healthy individuals. An abnormally high
  pressure is maintained only for short periods since the
  discomfort which arises from compression of tissues initiates
  changes in posture with consequent relief of pressure. Thus
  the limit of tolerance is rarely exceeded even in sleep, when
  positional changes occur 20–60 times during the night
- Movements are less frequent in patients who are
  - Severely ill or too weak to move
  - Suffering from paralysis, locomotor disorders or fractures
  - Drowsy or stuporose
  - In deep sleep due to heavy sedation
  - Undergoing long surgical operations
- Measurement of bodily movements during a 7-hour period
  at night has shown that a reduction in the number of
  movements is related to an increase in the number of
  pressure sores (Exton-Smith et al 1961). Approximately 80%
  of elderly in-patients make sufficient positional changes,
  but in 20% of cases the movements are inadequate and
  these patients are at risk of developing sores unless active
  preventive measures are taken
- The number of movements correlates with the general
  condition of the patient as assessed by the Norton score

Norton score

- A simple system can be used to assess the general condition
  of the patient and the severity of the illness
- The scores range from a maximum of 20 for the patient
  who is in physically good condition, mentally alert,
  ambulant, capable of full mobility and not incontinent, to a
  minimum of 5 for the patient in very bad physical state,
  stuporose, confined to bed, immobile and doubly incontinent
- There is an inverse relationship between the incidence of
  pressure sores and the Norton score at the time of
  admission to hospital
- The Norton score also determines the time at which
  pressure sores develop, and those with the lowest scores
  tend to develop sores during the early period of hospital

Table 29.1 Norton Score

Physical Condition	Mental State	Activity	Mobility	Incont	
Good	Alert	Ambulant	Full	Not	4
Fair	Apathetic	With help	Slightly limited	Occas.	3
Poor	Confused	Chairbound	Very limited	Usually	2
Very bad	Stuporose	Bedridden	Immobile	Doubly	1

stay. Approximately 70% of pressure sores in elderly patients occur in the first 2 weeks

Prevention

The majority of elderly patients admitted to a geriatric department are not particularly susceptible to the development of pressure sores and for them no special prophylactic measures are necessary. It is essential that the high-risk patients (20%) should be recognized.

Indentification of the patient at risk
— The Norton score should be used as a routine procedure in geriatric wards. Patients with a total score of 14 or less are liable to develop sores; the risk is very high when the score is less than 12
— The initial score is a reliable indicator in the majority of patients. For some patients, however, more frequent monitoring is needed since deterioration in general condition may not be recognized in time for the effective use of prophylactic measures

General measures
— There should be written instructions on the patient's basic needs so that all staff, especially the night nurses, understand the importance of maintaining effective preventive measures at all times
— The patient should be nursed mainly in bed, since bed-rest is important in the management of the patient whose severity of illness makes the development of pressure sores likely. The patient should be as flat as possible, allowing the weight to be distributed over a wide area and the application of anti-pressure measures
— The drawsheet should be soft and anchored under the pillow and at the sides to prevent wrinkling. A fleece helps to prevent friction over the sacral area and heels
— A bed-cradle should be used to take the weight of the bedclothes pressing on the feet
— The bed should be kept as dry as possible

— As soon as the general condition of the patient allows, early ambulation and the restoration of independent activity should be encouraged. These are beneficial in increasing mental alertness, restoring movement and increasing muscle tone. Patients who are able to sit in a chair should be encouraged to stand or at least lift themselves from the chair several times each hour

Regular turning

— Turning at 2-hourly intervals will reduce the incidence of pressure sores in the majority of patients at risk. It may, however, be difficult in some patients for whom it is most needed, e.g. in obese patients or those with contractures
— For seriously ill patients hourly turning may be required, but even this may fail to prevent tissue necrosis. Thus in many cases turning must be supplemented by anti-pressure devices

Preventing the adverse effects of direct pressure

Some of the more useful anti-pressure devices are

— Pillow beds consist of the positioning of pillows two or three thick to support the body, with gaps under bony prominences. Their effectiveness is limited in heavy, uncooperative or incontinent patients
— Soft foam mattresses are only partially effective owing to the difficulties in finding a suitable elastic water-proof covering material. The Polyflote mattress, made up of a double layer of foam with slits in the surface, is only effective without a cover
— The Vaperm mattress consists of sections of foam of varying densities and has an elastic vapour-permeable cover. It has properties which make it superior to the traditional mattress. It is generally acceptable to patients, but its effectiveness has not so far been assessed in clinical trials

Water mattresses

— True flotation beds, such as the Beaufort—Winchester, have a deep bath containing water at a controlled temperature with a loose envelope. The patient sinks into the water as if he were floating. The pressure is distributed over the whole of the undersurface of the body and there is no excess pressure over bony prominences
— Apart from the great nursing difficulties, water-beds are undoubtedly effective anti-pressure aids, but they are not appropriate for routine use in geriatric wards

Alternating pressure beds

— These mattresses have patterns of alternating air cells which are inflated and deflated by an electrically operated pump. The cycle of operation is 7–10 minutes, so that the points of

pressure on the undersurface of the body are continuously varied
— The large cell ripple mattress has been shown to be more effective than most other anti-pressure devices (Bliss et al 1967). Particular attention must be paid to the maintenance of the equipment.
— The Pegasus Air-Wave System is a development of the large cell ripple mattress and has a double layer of alternating pressure air cells. It has notable advantages. It is capable of preventing and healing sores even in patients who are not turned (Exton-Smith et al 1982). The inflating pressures are controlled automatically and are adjusted to the weight of the patient. Its effectiveness and reliability make it the most suitable equipment for preventing pressure sores in high-risk patients

Preventing shearing forces

Although many devices have been introduced to ameliorate the effects of direct compression, the problem of preventing tissue damage due to shearing forces has been relatively neglected.
— The water flotation bed completely eliminates shearing forces but it is extremely difficult to maintain the patient in a semi-upright position
— Raising the foot of the bed, with the patient nursed on an anti-pressure device, can be used to counteract the weight of the trunk which produces sliding; but it is difficult to obtain a correct balance in order to eliminate sliding completely

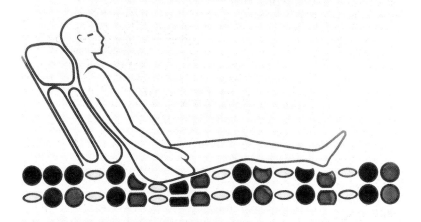

B cells inflated

Fig. 29.3 Pegasus Airwave System: contouring and the prevention of sliding.

— The Pegasus Air-Wave System has features which make it effective in reducing shearing forces over the sacral area. The contouring of the bed to the undersurface of the body when the patient is in the semi-recumbent position and the additional support given under the thighs prevent downward sliding (see Fig. 29.3). Even with the trunk inclined at 60° the proportion of the 7.5 min in which high pressure is sustained is about 15% and is well within the limits of tissue tolerance for intensity and duration of pressure.

Treatment of established sores

— Relief of pressure: the principle of pressure relief for the treatment of sores is the same as for prevention, but the anti-pressure measures must be applied more intensively. The Pegasus Air-Wave System is effective in promoting healing of sores. Superficial sores of the trunk heal quickly when relieved of pressure; deep sores take much longer to heal, often several months. Heel sores tend to be most intractable, since sloughs separate slowly and the healing process is prolonged by the poor vascularity and fixation of the surrounding tissue

— Local applications should be minimal. Antiseptics such as Eusol harm granulation and must not be used. Cavities should be washed out with normal saline and left empty. Packing with gauze and other material prevents discharge and contraction of the cavity with consequent prolongation of healing time and increase in pain

— Attention should be paid to the nutrition of the patient; in particular to the correction of negative nitrogen balance and the assessment of the vitamin C status. Zinc supplementation may be of help in promoting healing of pressure sores

BIBLIOGRAPHY

Barbenel J C, Jordon M M, Nicol S M, Clark M 1977 Incidence of pressure sores in the Greater Glasgow Health Board. Lancet 2: 548–550
Bliss M R, McLaren R, Exton-Smith A N 1967 Preventing pressure sores in hospital: A controlled trial of a large-celled ripple mattress. British Medical Journal 1: 394–397
Hibbs P, 1982 Pressure sores: A system of prevention. Nursing Mirror (4 August) 25–29
Exton-Smith A N, Overstall P W, Wedgwood J, Wallace G 1982 Use of an airwave system to prevent pressure sores in hospital. Lancet 1: 1288–1290
Exton-Smith A N, Sherwin R W 1961 The prevention of pressure sores: The significance of spontaneous bodily movements. Lancet 2: 1124–1126
Kosiak M 1961 Etiology of decubitus ulcers. Archives of Physical Medicine and Rehabilitation 42: 19–29
Norton D, McLaren R, Exton-Smith A N 1962 Investigation of geriatric nursing problems in hospital. National Corporation for the Care of Old People, London

30. HANDLING OF DRUGS AND IMPLICATIONS FOR PRESCRIBING

Adverse reactions

The growing elderly population is exposed to an increasing number and variety of drugs and is therefore at high risk from adverse drug reactions. These increase with age owing to the greater amount of medication prescribed for the elderly and their greater susceptibility to adverse reactions.

— Acknowledgement of the problems of medication in the elderly led to a special report by the Royal College of Physicians in 1984

— The higher incidence of polypharmacy in the elderly was reported by Moir & Dingwall-Fordyce (1980) in a study of drug-taking in people aged 65 years or over living at home. It was found that 28% had no medication, 57% had one to three prescribed drugs and 15% received four or more prescribed drugs

— A multicentre study reported by Williamson & Chopin (1980) found that more than 80% of elderly people admitted to departments of geriatric medicine in the UK were receiving prescribed medication. In 10% admission was completely or partly associated with an adverse drug reaction. The risk of adverse reactions was greatest with hypotensives (13.1%), followed by anti-parkinsonian drugs (13%), psychotropics (12.1%) and digitalis (11.5%). Table 30.1 lists drugs commonly prescribed to the elderly, with their main side effects. The prevalence of adverse reactions increased with the number of drugs being prescribed. The death rate due to this form of iatrogenic disease rises with age

Table 30.1 Drugs commonly prescribed to the elderly, with their main side effects

Drug	Side effects
Hypotensives	
Thiazide diuretics	Hypokalaemia
	Hyponatraemia
	Hypochloraemic alkalosis
	Hypercalcaemia
	Urinary incontinence
	Dehydration
	Dizziness
Beta-blockers[1]	Orthostatic hypotension
	Bronchospasm
	Depression
	Worsening of peripheral arterial disease
	Cardiac failure
	Impairment of psychomotor function
	Hyperglycaemia
Other hypotensives,	Dizziness
e.g. methyldopa,	Postural hypotension
prazosin, clonidine	Diarrhoea
Anti-parkinsonian drugs	Nausea and vomiting
e.g. levodopa, selegiline	Postural hypotension
	Confusional state
	Hallucination
Psychotropic drugs[2]	
Tricyclic antidepressants	Postural hypotension
	Cardiac arrythmias
	Urinary retention
Sedatives	Prolonged 'hangover' effect
	Confusion
	Postural hypotension
Digoxin	Nausea and vomiting
	Bradycardia
	Heartblock
	CNS disturbances,
	e.g. depression, memory impairment, delirium
Oral hypoglycaemic agents[3]	Prolonged hypoglycaemia

[1]Beta-blockers with high lipid solubility have a high incidence of side effects (especially CNS side effects) in the elderly and are best avoided, e.g. propranolol, oxprenolol, metoprolol.
[2]Use benzodiazepines with shorter half-lives, e.g. temazepam.
[3]Use agents with shorter duration of action, e.g. tolbutamide, glipizide.

Physiological changes

As people grow older there are a number of physiological changes, many of which influence the response of an individual to a given dose of a drug (Table 30.2). The main changes are
— Altered pharmacokinetics
— Altered pharmacodynamics
— Age-related physiological changes in body composition which affect drug handling

Table 30.2 Physiological changes affecting handling of drugs in the elderly

1. Absorption: unchanged

2. Distribution:
    Total body weight ↓
    Body water ↓   Drug concentration ↑
    Lean body mass ↓
    Body fat ↑ → Volume of distribution for highly
                lipid-soluble drugs ↑
    Plasma albumin ↓ → Protein-binding ↓ → Circulating free drug ↑

3. Elimination:
    Hepatic metabolism ↓
    Renal function ↓

4. Enhanced sensitivity, especially to CNS drugs

5. Impaired homeostasis

     — Drug-induced exacerbation of conditions which are common
        in the elderly

Altered pharmacokinetics
Age-related changes in drug absorption, distribution, metabolism and
excretion. The most important parameter in the aged patient is the rate
of elimination of a drug, which is mainly affected by the following:

Renal function
Both the glomerular filtration rate (GFR) and tubular secretion of drugs
decrease with age, leading to decreased renal drug excretion. Renal
blood flow and glomerular filtration rate fall by about 1% per annum
after the age of 30, so that by the eighth decade the GFR averages
60–80 ml/min. Therefore, drugs which are mainly excreted by the
kidneys should be prescribed in the lowest possible dose. They include:
acetazolamide, atenolol, captopril, cephalosporins, chlorpropamide,
cimetidine, digoxin, gentamicin, lithium, metformin, penicillins, ranitidine
and tolbutamide.

     — We recommend the use of the Siersbaek-Nielsen nomogram
        for rapid evaluation of endogenous creatinine clearance
        whenever this is necessary (Fig. 30.1)

     — Drugs with a narrow margin between safety and efficacy,
        i.e. a low therapeutic index, should also be prescribed in
        the lowest possible dose. They include digoxin,
        hypoglycaemic agents, lithium, phenytoin and
        anticonvulsants, theophylline and aminophylline. The patient
        should be seen regularly to screen for side effects and signs
        of overdose, and to monitor serum drug levels if necessary

Hepatic function
Hepatic blood flow decreases with age. Current evidence suggests that
most drugs which are extensively metabolized at the 'first pass' during
absorption from the gastrointestinal tract into the systemic circulation

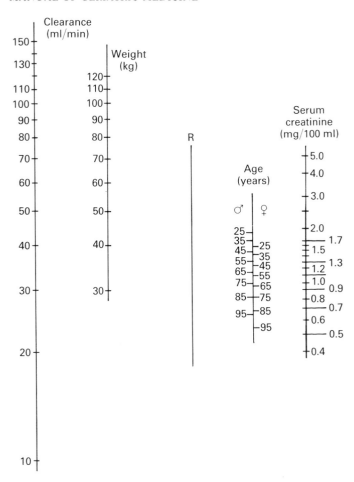

Fig. 30.1 Siersbaek-Nielsen nomogram: a nomogram for rapid evaluation of endogenous creatinine clearance. With a ruler, join weight to age. Keep ruler at crossing point of line marked R. Then move the right-hand side of the ruler to the appropriate serum creatinine value and read the patient's clearance from the left-hand side of the nomogram. From Kampmann et al 1974.

have a reduced rate of elimination and may therefore accumulate in the elderly. Drugs which are metabolized primarily by the liver include: chlormethiazole, isosorbide dinitrate, morphine derivatives, propranolol, salbutamol and verapamil.

Altered pharmacodynamics
Age-related changes in sensitivity to a given plasma and tissue drug concentration. Evidence suggests that in the elderly some drugs may produce an enhanced response for a given plasma concentration,

especially some drugs acting on the central nervous system such as benzodiazepines (e.g. diazepam, nitrazepam), digoxin, tricyclic antidepressants (e.g. amitriptyline, imipramine), warfarin.

Changes in body composition

Total body weight
This is reduced owing to an age-related reduction in intracellular water. This results in a decreased volume of distribution for highly water-soluble drugs (e.g. lithium).

Reduced muscle mass
This leads to a decreased volume of distribution for drugs which bind extensively to muscle (e.g. digoxin).

Increase in body fat
This leads to an increased volume of distribution for highly lipid-soluble drugs, especially in females (e.g. diazepam).

Reduced albumin levels
These occur especially in sick elderly patients. This can lead to decreased protein-binding of a drug, and therefore an increased proportion of the circulating free drug (e.g. thyroxine, warfarin, salicylates and non-steroidal anti-inflammatory drugs).

Exacerbation of existing conditions

Drugs can also exacerbate conditions which commonly occur in the elderly, such as

— Loss of postural stability leading to an increased incidence of falls: antihypertensives, diuretics, hypnotics and sedatives, vasodilators
— Constipation: antidepressants, anticholinergics, iron salts
— Hypothermia: phenothiazines, hypnotics and sedatives, antidepressants

Implications for prescribing

There are three main factors involved in the 'readiness to prescribe' to the elderly

1. The system of self-reporting of illness is not always adequate for the elderly, who may accept poor health as a consequence of ageing. Hence they may well consult their general practitioner only when a serious condition occurs. Such consultations frequently result in a prescription
2. In the very old, manifestations of normal ageing may be mistaken for disease and inappropriate medicines prescribed. A common misuse, for example, is the prescribing of prochlorperazine when an elderly person complains of vague giddiness due to impaired postural control
3. Multiple pathology may lead to polypharmacy

Medication regimen

This should be kept simple
  — Shorter treatment periods are preferable to prolonged therapy
  — Number of medications should be kept to a minimum; the elderly patient tends to make more mistakes when three or more concurrent medications are prescribed
  — Frequency of dosage should be kept to a minimum and one should try to give drugs as a single daily dose; if frequent dosage is necessary, administration of the drug(s) should be associated with daily routine such as mealtimes

Reduction of dosage

Due to the pharmacokinetic and pharmacodynamic changes occurring with age it is necessary as a general rule to reduce the dosage of drugs in the elderly. In aged patients treatment should be started at doses of little more than half that recommended for younger subjects. Paediatric formulations may provide greater flexibility of dose. The correct maintenance dose of a drug may be difficult to establish but is usually lower than for younger patients. Episodes of acute intercurrent illness may cause a rapid reduction in renal clearance, especially if there is concomitant dehydration, and therefore dosage must be reviewed and possibly reduced in these circumstances.

Review of medication

After the initial prescription the medication is not always reviewed. The elderly often find it difficult to visit surgeries owing to poor mobility, lack of transport, lack of an escort, fear of going out alone and especially of being attacked or mugged. Since they do not need illness certificates, there is no need for them to visit the general practitioner's surgery regularly. Consequently, there is a risk of multiple repeat prescriptions replacing consultations. Medication for the elderly should be reviewed both on a regular basis and in the event of an acute illness, so that drugs are kept to a minimum and discontinued whenever possible.

Compliance

Many studies have shown that medication prescribed does not equal medication taken. Patients deviate from their prescribed medication irrespective of age. Compliance is defined by Haynes as 'the extent to which the patient's behaviour coincides with medical or health advice'. A patient can be defined as non-compliant 'when the failure to comply is so significant as to interfere appreciably with achieving therapeutic goals'. The elderly often lack motivation to get better and consequently the level of non-compliance is higher. Therefore, it is important to give adequate explanations about the disease and the medication.

Patient counselling

This has been shown to improve compliance, and one study has found that 15 minutes' instruction with a pharmacist significantly reduced errors even in the poorly orientated. The doctor should explain the desired effect of the prescribed drug and should write clear instructions on the prescription. The patient should be instructed to report side effects.

Choice of preparations
This plays an important role in improving compliance. Liquid formulations are often more suitable than tablets. Poor compliance has been associated with changes in the formulations of drugs, and with variations in size, shape, colour or taste. Unpleasant or unacceptable side effects will promote non-compliance.

The container
This should be easy to open and should preferably be made of a transparent material such as plastic or glass, since many elderly patients recognize their medication by the shape, size and colour of the tablets. Child-resistant closures and foil-covered calendar packs are not recommended, for obvious reasons. A large 'palm-sized' traditional tablet bottle with an ordinary screw cap is the most suitable container in our experience. Some pharmaceutical companies have introduced special closures for arthritic hands.

    — Other types of containers which improve compliance are the 'Dosetts' and 'Medidos'. These are specially designed containers for patients on multiple drug regimens, which can be filled by patients, relatives, friends, district nurse or health visitor

The label
This should have clear instructions such as 'take one after breakfast, lunch and supper'. Instructions like bd, tds, nocte, prn, 'as directed' and 'as before' should be avoided. The purpose of the medication, e.g. 'heart', 'diabetes', 'blood pressure', will help the patient to remember the regimen. The instructions should be type-written, preferably in large print. For the partially sighted colour-coding of bottles or attaching matchsticks to containers (one matchstick for once per day) will improve compliance.

Memory aids
    — Specially designed containers, such as the 'Dosetts' and 'Medidos' and pill wheels, have been found to reduce the omission rate by up to 20%
    — They serve as a useful memory aid by helping the patient to know when to take the medicine; but they have the disadvantage of requiring weekly refilling and some elderly patients have found them awkward to handle. However, they are obviously better than 'egg cups' or 'egg trays', which leave the tablets exposed and are easily knocked over. For partially sighted patients the 'Dosett' box has instructions printed in Braille
    — Tablet identification cards and 'tear-off' calendars have been found to improve compliance only marginally

Supervision

Supervision of medication, if necessary, can be provided by relatives, friends, district nurse or health visitor. Hospitals should ensure that the elderly, on discharge, are properly counselled in the use of their medication and are given an adequate supply of drugs. Communication to the general practitioner should include details of the medication: dosage, frequency and duration of treatment. Domiciliary visits to review drug therapy could be made at regular intervals, e.g. by district nurse or health visitor, especially in the case of the elderly patient living alone. For patients in care or looked after by relatives, the reporting of untoward reactions or non-compliance should be encouraged. Patients should be asked to bring all their medicines when visiting the surgery or out-patient clinic. All discontinued treatment should be taken away from the patient, who may not feel inclined to throw away unrequired medicines.

BIBLIOGRAPHY

Adams K R H, Al-Hamouz S, Edmund E, Tallis R C, Vellodi C, Lye M 1987 Inappropriate prescribing in the elderly. Journal of the Royal College of Physicians of London 21: 39–41

Caird F I 1985 Towards rational drug therapy in old age. Journal of the Royal College of Physicians of London 19: 235–239

Coker N, Van der Cammen T J M 1987 Prescribing for the elderly: Pitfalls of therapy. Pulse Reference 47: 39–48

CSM Update 1985 Drugs and the elderly. British Medical Journal 1: 1345

Haynes R B 1979 In: Haynes R B, Taylor D W, Sacket D L (eds) Compliance in health care. John Hopkins University Press, Baltimore, pp 1–7

Kampmann J et al 1974 Acta Medica Scandinavica 196: 517–520

Moir D C, Dingwall-Fordyce T 1980 Drug taking in the elderly at home. Journal of Clinical and Experimental Gerontology 2: 329

Report of the Royal College of Physicians on Medication for the Elderly 1984. Journal of the Royal College of Physicians of London 18: 8–17

Siersbaek-Nielsen, Molholm Hansen J, Kampmann J, Kristensen M 1971 Rapid evaluation of creatinine clearance. Lancet 1: 1133–1134

Swift O G 1988 New Drugs: Prescribing in old age. British Medical Journal 2961: 913–915

Wandless I et al 1979 Compliance with prescribed medicines: A study of elderly patients in the community. Journal of the Royal College of General Practitioners 29: 391–396

Williamson J, Chopin J M 1980 Adverse reactions to prescribed drugs in the elderly: A multicentre investigation. Age and Ageing 9: 73–80

Index

Malnutrition *(contd)*
  definition, 159–160
  iatrogenic, 161
  prevalence, 160
  prevention, 171–172
  protein-energy, 163–165
  risk factors, 162–163
  vulnerable groups, 162
Mefenamic acid in osteoarthritis, 195
Memory impairment, drugs associated with, 213
Mental disturbances
  and malnutrition, 161
  in Parkinson's disease, 26
Mercury neuropathy, 175
Mesenteric ischaemia of small intestine, 115–116
Metabolic rate, 158
Metastatic bone disease, 188–189
Metered dose inhalers, 102–103
Methyldopa in hypertension, 69
Methyl prednisolone in osteoarthritis, 195
Metronidazole neuropathy, 175
Micturition syncope, 96
Midodrine in orthostatic hypotension, 95
Mitral valve disease, 87
Monoamine oxidase inhibitors, 51, 52
Multi-infarct dementia, 3, 37–38
  differential diagnosis with Alzheimer's disease, 42
Multiple myeloma, 138–139
Multiple sclerosis, urinary incontinence in, 259
Muscle, age changes in, 176–177
Muscle diseases, 176–182
  cramp, 181–182
  myasthenia gravis, 178–179
  myopathies, 177–178
  polymyalgia rheumatica, 180–181
  polymyositis, 179–180
Muscle relaxants in stroke, 14–15
Myasthenia gravis, 178–179
Mycoplasma, 100
Myelodysplastic syndrome, 134–135
Myocardial infarction, 76–80
  clinical features, 76–78
  complications of, 80
  diagnosis, 78–79
  management, 79–80
Myopathy, 177–178

Naproxen
  in gout, 203
  in osteoarthritis, 195
Neostigmine in myasthenia gravis, 178
Nephrotic syndrome, 128–129
Neuropathic arthropathy, 205
Neuropathy
  alcoholic, 174–175
  autonomic, 150
  diabetic, 149–150, 174
  drug-induced, 175
  and malignancy, 175
  vitamin B_{12} deficiency, 176
Neurotransmitters and depression, 48
Nifedipine
  in angina pectoris, 75–76
  in hypertension, 70–71

Nitrates
  in angina pectoris, 74–75
  in cardiac failure, 84
Nitrofurantoin neuropathy, 175
Nocturia, 56
Nocturnal leg movements, 55–56
Non-steroidal inflammatory drugs
  in gout, 203
  in osteoarthritis, 194–195
  in rheumatoid arthritis, 200
Noradrenaline disturbance in depression, 48
Nuclear magnetic resonance imaging in dementia, 41
Nutrients, recommended daily intake, 159
Nutrition, 158–173
  ascorbic acid deficiency, 168–170
  folate deficiency, 167–168
  iron deficiency *see* Anaemia, iron deficiency
  metabolic rate, 158
  recommended intakes of nutrients, 159
  vitamin B complex deficiency, 166–168
  vitamin D deficiency, 170–171
  see also Malnutrition

Ocular complications of diabetes mellitus, 149
Oesophageal candidiasis, 112–113
Oesophageal spasm, 112
Oesophagus, disorders of, 111–113
Orphenadrine in Parkinson's disease, 30
Orthostatic hypotension, 90–95
  aetiology, 91–93
  clinical features, 93
  definition, 90
  drug-induced, 91–92
  investigations, 93–94
  management, 94–95
  normal regulation of arterial pressure, 90
  in Parkinson's disease, 92
  pathophysiology, 90
  prevalence, 91
  see also Syncope
Osteoarthritis, 193–195
  clinical features, 193
  generalized, 194–195
Osteogenic sarcoma, 189–190
Osteomalacia, 185–187
  myopathy in, 177
Osteomyelitis, 190
  acute, 190–191
  chronic, 192
Osteoporosis, 183–185
Otitis externa, 238
Otitis media, 238–239
Ototoxicity, 243
Overflow incontinence, 258
Oxybutynin in urinary incontinence, 261

Pacemaker therapy, 86
Paget's disease of bone, 187–188
  affecting otic capsule, 243
Pain, 271–274
  anatomy and physiology, 271–272
  and sleep disturbance, 56
  treatment, 272–273